UPDATED AND EXPANDED
THIRD EDITION

EXCHANGES
FOR ALL
OCCASIONS

● ● ● ● ● ● ● ● ● ● ● ● ●

*How to Use the Exchange
System for Healthy and
Creative Food Choices*

● ● ● ● ● ● ● ● ● ● ● ● ●

MARION J. FRANZ, M.S., R.D., C.D.E.

**C H R O N I M E D
P U B L I S H I N G**
Minneapolis, Minnesota

Library of Congress Cataloging-in-Publication Data

Franz, Marion J.
Exchanges for all occasions./Marion J. Franz—[Updated and revised.]
p.   cm.
Includes bibliographical references and index.
ISBN 1-56561-005-9
1. Nutrition—Exchange Lists. 2. Diabetes—Popular works.
I. Franz, Marion J. II. International Diabetes Center. III. Title.

Editor: Peggy Linrud

Copy Editor and Indexing: Sylvia Timian

Cover and Text Design and Production: MacLean & Tuminelly

Illustrator: Jan Westberg

Printed in the United States of America

10 9 8 7 6 5

© 1983, revised 1987, 1993

International Diabetes Center
CHRONIMED Publishing
PO Box 47945
Minneapolis, MN 55447-9727

Exchange lists and nutritive values based on *Exchange Lists for Meal
Planning* © 1986, American Diabetes Association and The American
Dietetic Association.

▲ TABLE OF CONTENTS ▲

Part I   Expanded Exchange Lists

Part II   Exchanges for Special Occasions

Part III Guidelines for Food Purchasing and Preparation

Part IV Guidelines for Special Occasions

Tables

Sample Menus

▲ FOREWORD ▲

The original book, *Exchanges for All Occasions*, was published in 1982. It was written in response to the many questions asked on how to use exchange lists more effectively. It took several years (it was begun in 1979) to write the text in long hand, months to type and retype revisions, set in type, proofread again, and finally publish. This edition was written directly on a computer in six months, and the disk then edited, typeset, and printed. Such has been the change in the publication of books. The field of nutrition has also seen changes during the same period of time, but its importance in maintaining good health and reducing the chances of developing chronic diseases has remained constant—and even enhanced.

This new edition has been completely rewritten. The Food Guide Pyramid has been chosen as the theme because it illustrates the research-based food guidelines developed by the United States Department of Agriculture (USDA) with support by the Department of Health and Human Services (DHHS). The Pyramid helps you put Dietary Guidelines for Americans into action. The seven guidelines—eat a variety of foods; maintain healthy weight; choose a diet low in fat, saturated fat, and cholesterol; choose a diet with plenty of vegetables, fruits, and grain products; use sugars only in moderation; use salt and sodium only in moderation; and if you drink alcoholic beverages, do so in moderation—are the best, most up-to-date advice from nutrition scientists and are the basis of federal nutrition policy. The similarity between the Food Guide Pyramid and Exchange Lists is remarkable, emphasizing the point made in the original edition that nutritional recommendations for health are similar for all Americans.

This book has been written to help any of you who use exchange lists for planning your food intake to add variety, flexibility, and interest to your meal plans and to help health professionals with nutritional counseling. It is my hope this book will allow individuals to enjoy their meals and social life while still carefully following their meal plans.

A very special thanks to the wonderful and professionally skilled dietitians on the staff of the International Diabetes Center— Arlene Monk, Nancy Cooper, Broatch Haig, Barbara Barry, Gay Castle, Diane Reader, Betty Bajwa—for their ideas, editing suggestions, and support. Thanks also to Peggy Linrud and Sylvia Timian for their editing skills; to Nancy Tuminelly, art director, for her creative design; to Jan Westberg for her clever drawings; and to David Wexler, CHRONIMED, for his kind prodding which kept the book on track. Not to be forgotten is the entire IDC staff for their continued support and encouragement. They continue to be grand!

Marion J. Franz, MS, RD, CDE

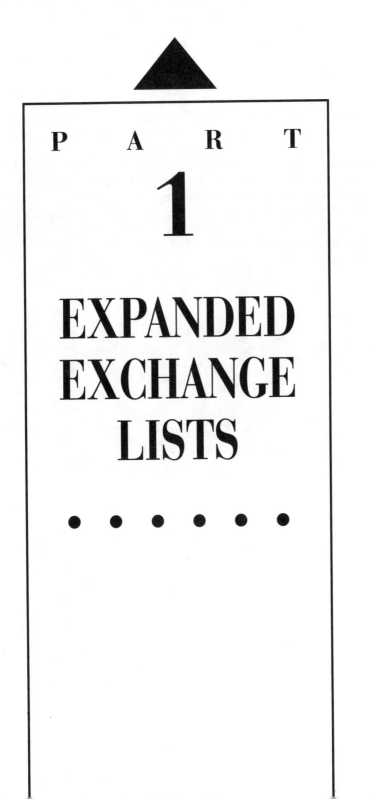

P A R T

1

EXPANDED EXCHANGE LISTS

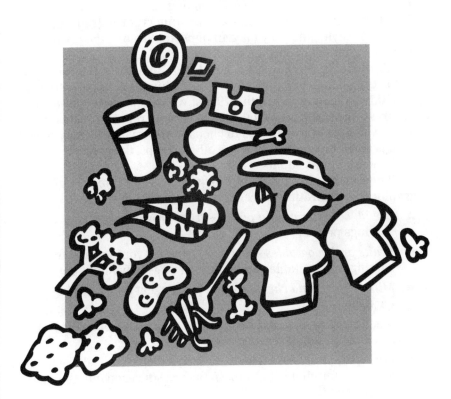

CHANGING THE SHAPE
OF NUTRITION

Many changes in the field of nutrition during the past two decades have altered old ways of thinking about food. Today, nutrition and exercise are recognized as important ingredients of a healthy lifestyle, and they play an important role in the prevention and management of chronic diseases.

To reflect these changes, a new Food Guide Pyramid, "erected" by the United States Department of Agriculture (USDA), is reshaping nutrition education. Since the 1950s, we've seen nutrition as four squares—the basic four food groups equally represented as quarters. Even if we were advised to choose two servings from two food groups and four servings from the other groups, the public tended to view the groups as equals.

The Food Guide Pyramid reorganizes food into five groups, graphically illustrating current nutrition guidelines.

▲ *Bread, cereal, rice and pasta*—great for you, so eat 6 to 11 servings per day.

▲ *Fruits and vegetables*—also very good for you, so eat 3 to 5 servings of vegetables and 2 to 4 servings of fruit per day.

▲ *Milk, yogurt, and cheese*—good for you, eat 2 to 3 servings each day.

▲ *Meat, poultry, fish, dry beans, eggs, and nuts*—okay for you, so eat 2 to 3 small servings each day.

▲ *Fats, oils, sweets*—can be trouble so eat sparingly; these foods are not a full-fledged group, so they're squeezed into the tip of the pyramid.

By placing grains at the bottom or foundation of the "eating right pyramid" (as it was originally called) and fruits, vegetables, meat and dairy products at levels above the grain group, the pyramid represents a totally new approach to nutrition education. The old guide simply advised variety in food choices but did not rank the importance of choices. Nor did the basic four recommend reducing fat intake.

Do the pyramid food groups remind you of the six exchange lists used for meal planning? Look at the pyramid food groups and substitute them with the exchange list groups. The base of the pyramid is the starch/bread exchange list, the fruit and vegetable exchange lists make up the next layer, and the meat and meat substitutes and milk exchange lists form a band near the top. Squeezed into the tip is the fat exchange list. The exchange lists point out how healthy the food choices are for you, your family and friends, and the public.

The food choices in the following chapters, based on the exchange lists and the Food Guide Pyramid, can help your food choices "stack up" in great shape.

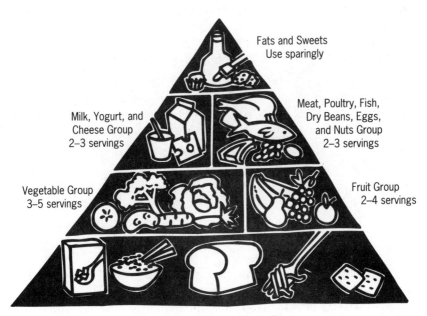

Fats and Sweets
Use sparingly

Milk, Yogurt, and
Cheese Group
2–3 servings

Meat, Poultry, Fish,
Dry Beans, Eggs,
and Nuts Group
2–3 servings

Vegetable Group
3–5 servings

Fruit Group
2–4 servings

Bread, Cereal, Rice, and Pasta Group
6–11 servings

Food Guide Pyramid
A Guide to Daily Food Choices

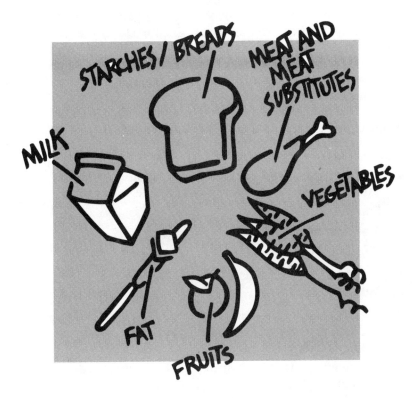

EASY MEAL PLANNING AND VARIETY WITH EXCHANGE LISTS

The exchange system has been developed to make meal planning easier for persons trying to control calories or for persons with diabetes. Exchange lists are based on the amount of carbohydrate, protein, fat, and calories in foods. Each exchange or choice has approximately the same number of calories and carbohydrate, protein, and fat content as other foods on the same list. Therefore, a food (in the amount listed) can be exchanged for any other food on the same list.

An "exchange" is a measured amount of food selected from a group of foods that is similar to it. *Exchange Lists for Meal Planning* was developed and published by The American Dietetic Association and the American Diabetes Association. It places foods into six groups (exchange lists), and the foods within a group have about the same nutritive value. Many foods fall into one of six groups:

▲ Starch/bread

▲ Meat and meat substitutes

▲ Vegetables

▲ Fruits

▲ Milk

▲ Fat

In addition to the six exchange lists of basic foods there are several other categories:

▲ Free foods—any food or drink with less than 20 calories per serving.

▲ Combination foods—foods such as casseroles, soups, and pizza, which contain foods from several lists.

▲ Special occasion foods—or the "dessert exchange list," including cake, cookies, ice cream, and simple desserts.

By using exchange lists you can select a variety of foods without calculating the value of each one. The "mix and match" or trade-off feature within the same food group makes it easier to select foods from a wider variety of foods, giving you more choices to "spice" up your daily fare.

A **meal plan** tells you how many servings you can select from each list for meals and snacks. Having a meal plan individualized for your calorie and lifestyle needs is important. Your meal plan helps you choose what and when you should eat throughout the day.

Exchange lists for many common foods are included in *Exchange Lists for Meal Planning* and are not all repeated here. The expanded exchange lists that follow apply the same principles to a greater variety of foods, making it easier to plan interesting and exciting meals.

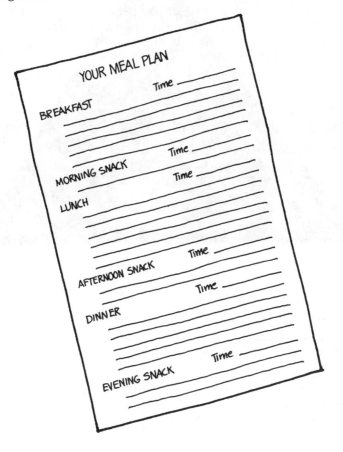

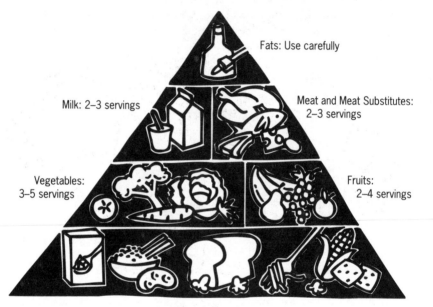

Fats: Use carefully

Milk: 2–3 servings

Meat and Meat Substitutes:
2–3 servings

Vegetables:
3–5 servings

Fruits:
2–4 servings

Starch/Bread:
6 or more servings

Exchange Lists

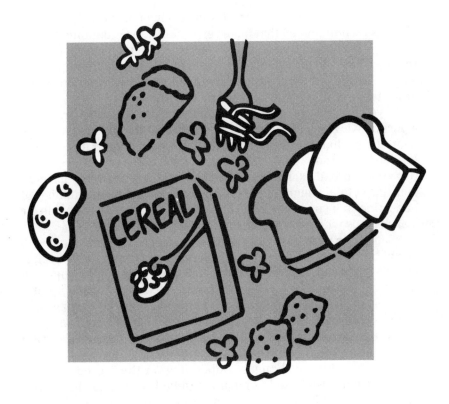

STARCH/BREAD
EXCHANGES

The base of the Food Guide Pyramid—and the first exchange list—contains breads, cereals, rice, and pasta—all foods from grains. You need to eat six to eleven servings of these foods each day. It's recommended that foods, especially those containing fiber, from this list be increased, while foods with fat and added sugars be reduced. Many of these foods are found on the starch/bread list. You will notice this is the first list, arranged to draw attention to the importance of these foods in your meal plan.

If you are unsure of the correct portion size for bread products, a portion weighing one ounce is a good rule of thumb. For example, a one-ounce hamburger or frankfurter bun or a one-ounce slice of French bread is one starch/bread exchange, and a two-ounce bun is two starch/bread exchanges. To tell if it is a one or two ounce bun, look at the total weight of the package and divide by the number of buns. One-half cup of cereal, grain, or pasta is another good rule for starch foods when you are unsure of the portion size.

Soups can most easily be counted as starch/bread exchanges. A cup of broth-type soup, such as chicken noodle or vegetable beef, is one starch/bread. A bowl of soup is usually closer to two cups and would be counted as two starch/bread exchanges. One cup of a cream soup is one starch/bread exchange plus one fat exchange.

Starch/bread and meat exchanges also can be used to count casseroles or mixed dishes. If you are unsure of the make up of a combination dish, count one cup as two starch/bread plus two medium fat meat exchanges. Depending on the ingredients the casserole may also include a fat or a vegetable exchange. For example, one cup of chili, beef stew, or macaroni and beef casserole is two starch/bread and two medium fat meat exchanges. One cup of tuna noodle casserole made with cream soup is one fat, two starch/bread and two medium fat meat exchanges.

General Guidelines for Starch/Breads

One Serving Equals:

1 ounce of a bread or snack product
¾ cup dry, unsweetened cereal
½ cup cooked cereal
4 to 5 snack crackers
½ cup pasta, starchy vegetable
⅓ cup rice, grains, stuffings
1 cup soup
½ cup cooked beans, peas, lentils
3 cups popcorn without added fat

▲ EXPANDED FOOD LIST ▲

Starch/Bread

Food value: The following foods contain approximately 15 grams of carbohydrate, 3 grams of protein, a trace of fat (about 1/2 to 1 gram), and 80 calories.

Whole grain breads, crackers, and grains such as kasha, couscous, bulgur, and wild rice average 2 grams of fiber per serving. Cereals containing fiber and starchy vegetables average 3 grams of fiber per serving. Bran cereals, dried beans, peas, and lentils will have 4 to 8 grams of fiber per serving.

FOOD	QUANTITY	EXCHANGES
Barley, cooked	⅓ cup	1 starch/bread
Beans:		
Baked beans, canned	⅓ cup	1 starch/bread

FOOD	QUANTITY	EXCHANGES
Baked beans, canned	1 cup	3 starch/bread 1 lean meat
Baked beans with franks, canned	½ cup	1 starch/bread 1 high fat meat
Beans, black, chickpeas, lentils, lima, mung, navy, pinto, cooked or canned	⅓ cup	1 starch/bread
Beans, black, chickpeas, lentils, lima, mung, navy, pinto, cooked or canned	1 cup	2 starch/bread 1 lean meat
Blackeyed peas, canned	⅓ cup	1 starch/bread
Cowpeas, frozen, boiled	⅓ cup	1 starch/bread
Dip, canned	¼ cup	1 starch/bread
Garbanzo beans, canned	⅓ cup	1 starch/bread
Peas, split, cooked	⅓ cup	1 starch/bread
Pork and beans in tomato sauce or pork 'n beans	⅓ cup	1 starch/bread
Refried beans	½ cup	1½ starch/bread ½ lean meat
Soybeans, cooked	½ cup	½ starch/bread 1 med. fat meat
Breads:		
Bagel	½ (1 oz.)	1 starch/bread
Baking powder or buttermilk biscuits	1	1 starch/bread 1 fat
Banana bread	1 slice (1⁄16 loaf)	1 starch/bread 1 fat
Boston brown bread	1 slice (3" round x ½")	1 starch/bread
Bread crumbs, dry	3 Tbsp.	1 starch/bread
Bread, home baked or unsliced	1 oz.	1 starch/bread
Bread sticks, 8" long, ½" diameter	2	1 starch/bread
Bread sticks, 4" long, ¼" diameter	6	1 starch/bread
Brown and Serve rolls	1 average	1 starch/bread
Corn bread	2" square	1 starch/bread 1 fat

FOOD	QUANTITY	EXCHANGES
Corn pone	1 cake (1½ oz.)	1 starch/bread ½ fat
Crescents or twists	1 roll	1 starch/bread 1 fat
Croissants	1 average	1½ starch/bread 2½ fat
Croissants, petite	1	1 starch/bread 1½ fat
Croutons	⅔ cup	1 starch/bread
Crumpet	1	1 starch/bread
Diet bread (40 calories/slice)	2	1 starch/bread
Dinner rolls	1 average	1 starch/bread
English muffins, all varieties	1	2 starch/bread
French bread	3" slice	1 starch/bread
French toast	1 slice	1 starch/bread ½ med fat meat
Hard rolls	1	1½ starch/bread
Muffins, banana nut, blueberry, apple cinnamon	1 small	1 starch/bread 1 fat
Muffins, carrot nut, chocolate chip, oatmeal raisin	1 small	1½ starch/bread 1 fat
Muffins, oat bran, streusel varieties	1 small	1½ starch/bread 1½ fat
Muffins, light	1 average	1 starch/bread
Muffins, hearty style	1	2 starch/bread 1½ fat
Party breads (pumpernickel, rye)	4 slices	1 starch/bread
Patty shell	1	1 starch/bread 3 fat
Pocket or pita bread, 4½" diameter	1	1 starch/bread
Pocket or pita bread, 6½" diameter	½ loaf (1 oz.)	1 starch/bread
Popover	1 small	1 starch/bread 1 fat
Rice cakes, all varieties	2 cakes	1 starch/bread
Rice cakes, mini	½ oz.	1 starch/bread
Spoon bread	3½ oz.	1 starch/bread 2 fat
Taco shells	2	1 starch/bread 1 fat

FOOD	QUANTITY	EXCHANGES
Tea breads (pumpkin, cranberry, etc.)	1 slice (1½ oz.)	1½ starch/bread 1 fat
Tortillas, corn	1	1 starch/bread
Tortillas, flour, 8"	1	1 starch/bread
Tortillas, flour, 10"	1	1½ starch/bread
Tortillas, flour, 12"	1	2 starch/bread
Tostada shells	2	1 starch/bread 1 fat
Buckwheat groats (kasha), cooked	½ cup	1 starch/bread
Bulgur, cooked	½ cup	1 starch/bread
Carob flour, (St. Johnsbread)	2 tablespoons	1 starch/bread
Cereals:		
Ready-to-Eat Cereals		
All Bran	⅓ cup	1 starch/bread
All Bran with Extra Fiber	¾ cup	1 starch/bread
Apple Raisin Crisp	⅔ cup	1 starch/bread 1 fruit
Bran Buds	⅓ cup	1 starch/bread
Bran Chex	½ cup	1 starch/bread
Bran Flakes	⅔ cup	1 starch/bread
40% Bran	½ cup	1 starch/bread
100% Bran	⅓ cup	1 starch/bread
Cheerios	1 cup	1 starch/bread
Cheerios, Apple Cinnamon, Honey Nut	½ cup	1 starch/bread
Corn Bran	½ cup	1 starch/bread
Corn Chex	¾ cup	1 starch/bread
Corn Flakes	¾ cup	1 starch/bread
Crispy Wheats 'n Raisins	¾ cup	1 starch/bread ½ fruit
Fiber One	½ cup	1 starch/bread
Fruit and Fibre	⅓ cup	1 starch/bread
Fruit Muesli, all varieties	½ cup	1 starch/bread 1 fruit
Granola	¼ cup	1 starch/bread ½ fat
Grape Nuts	3 tablespoons	1 starch/bread
Grape Nuts Flakes	⅔ cup	1 starch/bread 1 fat

FOOD	QUANTITY	EXCHANGES
Kix	1 cup	1 starch/bread
Life	⅔ cup	1 starch/bread
Mueslix Crispy Blend	⅔ cup	1 starch/bread 1 fruit ½ fat
Mueslix Golden Crunch	½ cup	1 starch/bread ½ fruit
Nutri-Grain Almond Raisin	⅔ cup	1 starch/bread 1 fruit
Nutri-Grain Raisin Bran	1 cup	1 starch/bread 1 fruit
Nutri-Grain Wheat	½ cup	1 starch/bread
Oat Bran	½ cup	1 starch/bread
Oatmeal Crisp	¾ cup	1 starch/bread
Puffed Rice	1½ cup	1 starch/bread
Puffed Wheat	1½ cup	1 starch/bread
Raisin Bran	½ cup	1 starch/bread
Raisin Nut Bran	½ cup	1 starch/bread ½ fat
Raisin Oat Bran	¾ cup	1 starch/bread 1 fruit
Rice Chex	¾ cup	1 starch/bread
Rice Krispies	¾ cup	1 starch/bread
Sunflakes Multi Grain	¾ cup	1 starch/bread
Shredded Wheat	1 biscuit	1 starch/bread
Shredded Wheat Squares	½ cup	1 starch/bread
Special K	¾ cup	1 starch/bread
Team Flakes	¾ cup	1 starch/bread
Total	¾ cup	1 starch/bread
Total Raisin Bran	1 cup	1 starch/bread 1 fruit
Wheat Chex	½ cup	1 starch/bread
Wheaties	¾ cup	1 starch/bread
Hot Cereals, Cooked		
Corn Grits	½ cup	1 starch/bread
Corn Meal	⅓ cup	1 starch/bread
Cream of Rice	½ cup	1 starch/bread
Cream of Wheat	½ cup	1 starch/bread
Farina	¾ cup	1 starch/bread
Grits, Instant, Plain	1 pkt.	1 starch/bread

FOOD	QUANTITY	EXCHANGES
Grits, Instant, All Flavors	1 pkt.	1 starch/bread
Malt-O-Meal	⅔ cup	1 starch/bread
Maypo	½ cup	1 starch/bread
Oat Bran	⅓ cup	1 starch/bread
Oatmeal, Quick and Old Fashioned	⅔ cup	1 starch/bread
Oatmeal, Instant, Regular	1 pkt.	1 starch/bread
Oatmeal, Instant, Flavored	1 pkt.	2 starch/bread
Ralston	⅔ cup	1 starch/bread
Roman Meal	½ cup	1 starch/bread
Wheatena	½ cup	1 starch/bread
Chapati, 5" to 6" diameter	1	1 starch/bread 1 fat
Cornstarch	2 Tbsp.	1 starch/bread
Couscous, cooked	⅓ cup	1 starch/bread
Crackers:		
Animal	7	1 starch/bread
American Classic, all varieties	8	1 starch/bread 1 fat
Cheese-filled crackers	6 (1.5 oz.)	1½ starch/bread 2 fat
Cheese Nips	20	1 starch/bread 1 fat
Club	8	1 starch/bread 1 fat
Goldfish crackers, all varieties	45	1 starch/bread 1 fat
Harvest Crisp, all varieties	12	1 starch/bread 1 fat
Matzo, 6" diameter	1 (¾ oz.)	1 starch/bread
Matzo crackers, 1½" sq.	7	1 starch/bread
Meal Mates Wafers	5 average	1 starch/bread 1 fat
Melba toast, long	5	1 starch/bread
Melba toast, rounds	8	1 starch/bread
Oat Bran Krisp crackers	4 triple	1 starch/bread 1 fat
Oyster, large	30	1 starch/bread
Oyster, small	60	1 starch/bread

FOOD	QUANTITY	EXCHANGES
Peanut-butter filled crackers	6 (1.5 oz.)	1½ starch/bread 2 fat
Ritz, Hi Ho, etc.	6	1 starch/bread 1 fat
Rusk	2	1 starch/bread
RyKrisp, all varieties	4 triple crackers	1 starch/bread
Snack Sticks, all varieties	8	1 starch/bread 1 fat
Sociables	8	1 starch/bread 1 fat
Toasted Snack, all varieties	8	1 starch/bread 1 fat
Town House	8	1 starch/bread 1½ fat
Triscuit wafers	6	1 starch/bread 1 fat
Uneeda biscuits	5	1 starch/bread 1 fat
Waverly wafers	6	1 starch/bread 1 fat
Wheat Thins	14	1 starch/bread 1 fat
Zweibach	3 (¾ oz.)	1 starch/bread
Falafel, 2" diameter patties	3 patties	1 starch/bread 1 med.fat meat 2 fat
Farfel, dry	3 Tbsp.	1 starch/bread
Flour	3 Tbsp.	1 starch/bread
Hominy, cooked	½ cup	1 starch/bread
Hummus	⅓ cup	1 starch/bread 1½ fat
Miso	½ cup	2½ starch/bread 1 med.fat meat
Noodles, cellophane	¾ cup	1 starch/bread
Noodles, chow mein	⅓ cup	1 starch/bread
Pancakes, frozen or microwave, 4" cakes	3	2½ starch/bread 1 fat
Polenta	⅓ cup	1 starch/bread
Quinoa, cooked	⅓ cup	1 starch/bread

FOOD	QUANTITY	EXCHANGES
Rice:		
Basmati aromatic rice	½ cup	1 starch/bread
Brown, cooked	⅓ cup	1 starch/bread
Rice, fried	½ cup	1 starch/bread
		2 fat
Rice, instant, cooked	⅓ cup	1 starch/bread
Rice, long-grain, cooked	⅓ cup	1 starch/bread
Sauces:		
Cheese, prepared with milk	½ cup	1 starch/bread
		1 high fat meat
Spaghetti sauce	½ cup	1 starch/bread
Spaghetti, chunky	½ cup	1 starch/bread
Stroganoff, prepared with	½ cup	1 starch/bread
milk and water		1 fat
Scrapple	2 slices	1 starch/bread
		1 high fat meat
Snack Foods:		
Bugles,	30	1 starch/bread
all varieties	(1 oz.)	1½ fat
Cheetos,	1 oz.	1 starch/bread
all varieties		2 fat
Cheetos, light	1 oz.	1 starch/bread
		1 fat
Chex Snack Mix,	⅔ cup	1 starch/bread
all varieties	(1 oz.)	1 fat
Dinosaur Grahams	1 large	1 starch/bread
Doo Dads	½ cup	1 starch/bread
	(1 oz.)	1 fat
Doritos tortilla chips,	15–18 chips	1 starch/bread
all varieties	(1 oz.)	1 fat
Doritos light tortilla	1 oz.	1 starch/bread
chips, all varieties		1 fat
Fritos corn chips,	~34 chips	1 starch/bread
all varieties	(1 oz.)	2 fat
Granola bars,	1 bar	1 starch/bread
all varieties		1 fat
Party Mix	¼ cup	1 starch/bread
		2 fat
Popcorn, hot air	5 cups	1 starch/bread

FOOD	QUANTITY	EXCHANGES
Popcorn, microwave popped	3 cups	1 starch/bread 2 fat
Popcorn, microwave, light popped	5 cups	1 starch/bread 1 fat
Potato chips	1 oz.	1 starch/bread 2 fat
Pretzels	¾ oz.	1 starch/bread
Very thin twisted	4	1 starch/bread
Pretzelettes	12	1 starch/bread
Very thin sticks	65	1 starch/bread
Sesame chips	¼ cup	1 starch/bread 2 fat
Teddy Grahams	15	1 starch/bread ½ fat
Somen or udon (noodles), cooked	⅓ cup	1 starch/bread
Soups, canned or dehydrated:		
Cream of asparagus, prepared with water	1 cup	1 starch/bread 1 fat
Bean, black, prepared with water	1 cup	1 starch/bread
Bean with bacon, prepared with water	1 cup	1½ starch/bread 1 fat
Bean with ham, chunky	1 cup	2 starch/bread 1 med.fat meat
Beef, chunky	1 cup	1 starch/bread 1 med.fat meat
Beef noodle, prepared with water	1 cup	1 starch/bread
Cheese, prepared with water	1 cup	1 starch/bread 2 fat
Chicken, chunky	1 cup	1 starch/bread 1 med.fat meat
Chicken noodle, prepared with water	1 cup	1 starch/bread
Chicken rice, prepared with water	1 cup	1 starch/bread
Chili beef, prepared with water	1 cup	1½ starch/bread 1 fat
Clam chowder, Manhattan, prepared with water	1 cup	1 starch/bread

FOOD	QUANTITY	EXCHANGES
Clam chowder, New England, prepared with milk	1 cup	1 starch/bread 1 fat
Lentil with ham	1 cup	1½ starch/bread 1 fat
Minestrone, chunky	1 cup	1½ starch/bread
Minestrone, prepared with water	1 cup	1 starch/bread
Cream of mushroom, prepared with water	1 cup	1 starch/bread 1 fat
Oyster stew, prepared with milk	1 cup	1 starch/bread 1 fat
Pea, split, with ham, chunky	1 cup	1½ starch/bread 1 lean meat
Pea, split, with ham, prepared with water	1 cup	2 starch/bread 1 lean meat
Potato, cream of, prepared with water	1 cup	1 starch/bread 1 fat
Ramen noodle, all varieties as prepared	1 pkg. (2.19 oz.)	2½ starch/bread 1½ fat
Ramen noodle, low fat	1 pkg.	3 starch/bread
Tomato bisque, prepared with water	1 cup	1½ starch/bread
Tomato, prepared with with water	1 cup	1 starch/bread
Tomato rice, prepared with water	1 cup	1½ starch/bread
Turkey, chunky	1 cup	1 starch/bread 1 med.fat meat
Turkey noodle, prepared with water	1 cup	1 starch/bread
Vegetable, chunky	1 cup	1 starch/bread 1 fat
Vegetable, vegetarian, prepared with water	1 cup	1 starch/bread
Vegetable with beef	1 cup	1 starch/bread
Won ton soup, canned	1 cup	½ starch/bread
Starchy Vegetables:		
Chestnuts	4 large, 6 small	1 starch/bread
Corn, canned	½ cup	1 starch/bread

FOOD	QUANTITY	EXCHANGES
Corn, sweet	I med. ear	1 starch/bread
Corn, cream style	⅓ cup	1 starch/bread
Corn pudding	½ cup	1 starch/bread 1 fat
Eggplant, cooked	2 cups 1" cubes	1 starch/bread
Malanga, boiled	⅓ cup	1 starch/bread
Mixed vegetables	¾ cup	1 starch/bread
Onion rings, frozen	4 rings	1 starch/bread 2 fat
Parsnips, cooked	½ cup, sliced	1 starch/bread
Peas, green, cooked	½ cup	1 starch/bread
Peas and carrots, cooked	¾ cup	1 starch/bread
Peas and onions, cooked	1 cup	1 starch/bread
Poi, (taro, cooked)	⅓ cup	1 starch/bread
Potatoes:		
Au gratin, home-prepared	½ cup	1 starch/bread 2 fat
Au gratin, mix, prepared	½ cup	1 starch/bread 1 fat
French-fried, frozen, heated in oven	10 strips	1 starch/bread 1 fat
French-fried, frozen, restaurant-prepared	10 strips	1 starch/bread 2 fats
Hash brown	½ cup	1 starch/bread 2 fat
Potatoes O'Brien	½ cup	1 starch/bread
Potato chips	15 chips	1 starch/bread 2 fat
Potato pancakes	1	2 starch/bread 2 fat
Potato puffs, frozen, prepared	½ cup	1 starch/bread 1 fat
Potato salad	½ cup	1 starch/bread 2 fat
Scalloped	½ cup	1 starch/bread 1 fat
Stix or shoestrings	¾ cup (1 oz.)	1 starch/bread 2 fat

FOOD	QUANTITY	EXCHANGES
Tater-Tots	½ cup	1 starch/bread 1 fat
Twice-baked, frozen	1 (5 oz.)	2 starch/bread 2 fat
Rutabaga, mashed	¾ cup	1 starch/bread
Salsify or oyster plant	¾ cup	1 starch/bread
Succotash	½ cup	1 starch/bread
Sweet potato, mashed	⅓ cup	1 starch/bread
Sweet potato	½ med.	1 starch/bread
Yam, cubes, cooked	½ cup	1 starch/bread
Spaetzle	⅓ cup	1 starch/bread
Stuffings:		
Stuffing mix, all varieties, as prepared	⅓ cup	1 starch/bread 1 fat
Stuffing mix, microwave	⅓ cup	1 starch/bread 1 fat
Tapioca, dry	2 Tbsp.	1 starch/bread
Tempeh	½ cup	1 starch/bread 2 lean meats
Waffles:		
Waffles, frozen, all varieties	1	1 starch/bread 1 fat
Miniature	4 mini	1 starch/bread ½ fat
Nutri-Grain, frozen, all varieties	1	1 starch/bread 1 fat
Wheat Germ, toasted, plain	¼ cup	1 starch/bread 1 lean meat
Wild Rice, cooked	½ cup	1 starch/bread

Word List

Bulgur: Whole wheat berry that is parboiled, dried, and broken up. Cooks very quickly.

Carob: A long, edible sweet pod that grows on an evergreen tree in the Mediterranean region. It has a flavor like milk chocolate. The pod can be ground and used in baked products. It is also called carob bean, honey bread, or locust bean.

Cassava: Also known as the yucca root. It has a large, starchy root. The starch derived from the root of this plant is used to make tapioca. It has a bitter odor that disappears with cooking.

Chapati: A thin, grilled, pancake-shaped whole wheat bread, popular in Indian cookery, made with or without fat.

Chestnuts: A nut that has a hard, brown outer shell and an inner shell that protects the kernel. To shell, make a deep x on the flat side; cover with boiling water, and simmer 2 to 3 minutes; drain 2 to 3 nuts at a time; and pull off shells and inner skins. To roast, make a deep x on flat side; roast in a fireplace, place nuts on edge of open fire or in a long-handled popcorn basket. Shake over fire until they pop.

Couscous: Precooked hard-cracked granules of semolina wheat. It can be cooked quickly by a soak and steam method.

Falafel: Patties made from coarse-ground wheat germ, garbanzo beans, fava beans, and spices and then lightly fried in oil.

Farfel: Noodle dough grated into barley-sized grains and served in soup.

Malanga: A starchy white tuber grown in the tropics for the edible root.

Quinoa: A tiny, millet-like seed used as a grain, originally from South America. It has a delicate flavor with a couscous-like texture. Before cooking, always rinse the grain well to remove a slightly bitter coating.

Salsify: Also known as vegetable oyster or oyster plant. It is a grassy, flat, green plant with pale tan flesh and an oyster flavor.

Spaetzle: A German side dish served in place of potatoes or rice and often accompanied by a sauce or gravy. It is made from flour, eggs, and water or milk, formed into tiny noodles or dumplings by either rolling the dough or forcing it through a sieve, and then usually boiled.

Succotash: A dish of North American Indian origin consisting of corn and beans.

Taro root: Also known as dasheen, tannia, eddo, malanga, and tannier. It has a brown shaggy covering and white, creamy flesh. Commonly used in Hawaii and eaten in the form of poi. Cooked taro ranges in color from purple to cream.

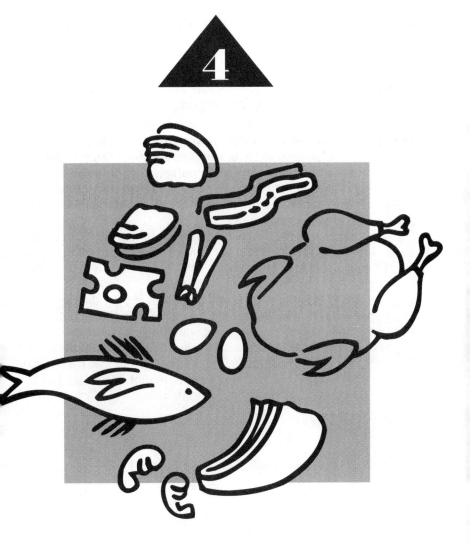

MEAT AND MEAT SUBSTITUTES EXCHANGES

Meats are the third layer of the Food Guide Pyramid but the second exchange list. This is because in meal planning the meat and starch food choices are often the main entrees. However, meats should be treated more as an accompaniment to the starch and vegetable choices and not as the main entree. Two to three servings consisting of two to three ounces of cooked lean meat, poultry, or fish or servings of cooked dried beans, eggs, or nuts such as peanut butter are recommended daily.

Meat portion sizes are based on cooked meat with the fat and bones removed. Because meat portions are difficult to estimate, it is helpful to weigh meat. This is especially important when preparing meats you have not used before.

You can help reduce the total fat content of your diet by choosing leaner cuts of meat, using food preparation methods that eliminate fat in the cooking process, and watching your portion sizes.

Meat is divided into three categories to help you identify the fat content: lean meat, medium-fat meat, and high-fat meat. The foods listed contain approximately the same amount of protein but are divided into three lists based on fat content.

▲

General Guidelines for Meat and Meat Substitutes

One exchange equals:
1 ounce meat, fish, poultry
1 ounce cheese
1 egg

Average serving = 3 meat exchanges:
3 ounce portion of meat (about
the size of a deck of playing cards)

Lean meat choices:
Fish, poultry, lean beef (round,
sirloin, flank steak), processed hams, veal,
cottage cheese, low-fat cheeses,
lean luncheon meats

Medium-fat meat choices:
Most beef and pork, poultry with skin,
skim milk cheeses, eggs

High-fat meat choices:
Fried meats, poultry, or fish; prime
cuts of beef, corned beef, spareribs,
regular cheeses, regular luncheon meats,
sausages, hot dogs, peanut butter

▲ EXPANDED FOOD LIST ▲

Lean Meat

Food value: The following foods contain approximately 7 grams of protein, 3 grams of fat, and 55 calories. Each is equal to one lean meat exchange.

FOOD	QUANTITY	EXCHANGES
Beef:		
Beef jerky	½ oz.	1 lean meat
Chuck, arm pot roast	1 oz.	1 lean meat
Dried chipped beef	1 oz.	1 lean meat
Eye of round	1 oz.	1 lean meat
Family steak	1 oz.	1 lean meat
Filet mignon	1 oz.	1 lean meat
Flank steak	1 oz.	1 lean meat
Kabob cubes	1 oz.	1 lean meat
Loin top	1 oz.	1 lean meat
London broil	1 oz.	1 lean meat
Round bottom	1 oz.	1 lean meat
Round tip roast	1 oz.	1 lean meat
Round top steak	1 oz.	1 lean meat
Shank	1 oz.	1 lean meat
Sirloin steak	1 oz.	1 lean meat
Skirt steak	1 oz.	1 lean meat
Stew meat	1 oz.	1 lean meat
Sweetbreads	1 oz.	1 lean meat
Tenderloin	1 oz.	1 lean meat
Tenderloin steak	1 oz.	1 lean meat
Tenderloin tips	1 oz.	1 lean meat
Top sirloin	1 oz.	1 lean meat
Very lean ground round or sirloin (90% lean)	1 oz.	1 lean meat
Cheese:		
Alpine Lace Free 'n Lean cheese products, cheddar, mozzarella, cream cheese, cheese spread	1 oz.	1 lean meat

FOOD	QUANTITY	EXCHANGES
Borden Lite-Line American, mild and sharp cheddar, Colby, Monterey Jack, mozzarella, Swiss	1 oz.	1 lean meat
Cottage cheese	¼ cup	1 lean meat
Cottage cheese 1%	¼ cup	1 lean meat
Cottage cheese 2%	¼ cup	1 lean meat
Fisher Countdown cheese spread	1 oz.	1 lean meat
Kaukauna Lite 50 cold pack cheese product	1 oz.	1 lean meat
Kraft light and nonfat singles pasteurized process cheese product	1 oz.	1 lean meat
Laughing Cow reduced calorie	1 oz.	1 lean meat
Lifetime fat free pasteurized process cheese, natural part skim milk cheese	1 oz.	1 lean meat
Ricotta natural part skim	1 oz. (2 tbsp.)	1 lean meat
Sargento		
Pot cheese	1½ oz.	1 lean meat
Ricotta lite	2 oz.	1 lean meat
Weight Watchers process cheese product, all varieties	1 oz.	1 lean meat
Weight Watchers (reduced calorie) cream cheese	1 oz.	1 lean meat
Eggs:		
Egg whites	2	1 lean meat
Egg substitute	¼ cup	1 lean meat
Fish:		
Blue crab, steamed	1½ oz.	1 lean meat
Catfish, baked	1 oz.	1 lean meat
Clam, steamed	4 small	1 lean meat
Cod, broiled	1½ oz.	1 lean meat
Crab Dungeness	1½ oz.	1 lean meat
Crab meat, canned	¼ cup	1 lean meat
Crab cakes	1	2 lean meat
Crayfish	16	1 lean meat

FOOD	QUANTITY	EXCHANGES
Flounder, baked	1½ oz.	1 lean meat
Frog legs	3 medium	1 lean meat
Haddock, baked	1½ oz.	1 lean meat
Halibut, broiled	1 oz.	1 lean meat
Lobster	1½ oz.	1 lean meat
Mussels	2 oz.	1 lean meat
Ocean perch, baked	1½ oz.	1 lean meat
Octopus	1 oz.	1 lean meat
Orange roughy, broiled	2 oz.	1 lean meat
Oyster, steamed	5 medium	1 lean meat
Pollock, broiled	1½ oz.	1 lean meat
Rainbow trout, broiled	1 oz.	1 lean meat
Rockfish, baked	1½ oz.	1 lean meat
Salmon, Atlantic/coho	1 oz.	1 lean meat
Scallops, broiled	2 large or 5 small	1 lean meat
Shrimp, boiled	1½ oz.	1 lean meat
Smelt	1 oz.	1 lean meat
Sole, broiled	1½ oz.	1 lean meat
Squid	1 oz.	1 lean meat
Trout	1 oz.	1 lean meat
Tuna, light, canned	1 oz.	1 lean meat
Tuna, yellowfin, broiled	1 oz.	1 lean meat
Walleye pike	1½ oz.	1 lean meat
Whiting, baked	1½ oz.	1 lean meat
Game:		
Buffalo	1 oz.	1 lean meat
Rabbit, roasted	1 oz.	1 lean meat
Squirrel, roasted	1 oz.	1 lean meat
Venison, roasted	1 oz.	1 lean meat
Lamb:		
Cubes, stew	1 oz.	1 lean meat
Shish kabob	1 oz.	1 lean meat
Shoulder roast	1 oz.	1 lean meat
Sirloin roast	1 oz.	1 lean meat
Pork:		
Boiled ham	2 slices	1 lean meat
Boneless loin roast	1 oz.	1 lean meat
Boneless rib roast	1 oz.	1 lean meat
Boneless sirloin chop	1 oz.	1 lean meat

FOOD	QUANTITY	EXCHANGES
Boneless smoked ham, (95% lean)	1 oz.	1 lean meat
Boneless top loin chop	1 oz.	1 lean meat
Canadian-style bacon	1 oz.	1 lean meat
Canned or cured hams	1 oz.	1 lean meat
Center loin chop	1 oz.	1 lean meat
Rib chop	1 oz.	1 lean meat
Sirloin roast	1 oz.	1 lean meat
Tenderloin	1 oz.	1 lean meat
Poultry:		
Capon	1 oz.	1 lean meat
Chicken, diced	¼ cup	1 lean meat
Chicken giblets or gizzard	1 oz.	1 lean meat
Chicken livers, simmered	4 average	1 lean meat
Chicken, canned	1 oz.	1 lean meat
Pheasant	1 oz.	1 lean meat
Quail	1 oz.	1 lean meat
Squab (pigeon)	1 oz.	1 lean meat
Smoked turkey breast	1 oz.	1 lean meat
Turkey ham	1 oz.	1 lean meat
Processed Meats:		
Cold cuts (95% or more fat free)	2 slices	1 lean meat
Corned beef loaf, jellied	1 oz.	1 lean meat
Franks, Hormel Light & Lean, Healthy Choice, or Healthy Favorites	1	1 lean meat
Thin sliced meats: beef, chicken, corned beef, ham, turkey	1 oz. (5 slices)	1 lean meat
Turkey lunch meats: roasted breast, ham, pastrami	1 oz. (1 slice)	1 lean meat
Veal:		
Chop, loin or rib	1 oz.	1 lean meat
Cubes for kabobs	1 oz.	1 lean meat
Cutlet	1 oz.	1 lean meat
Roast	1 oz.	1 lean meat
Steak cutlet	1 oz.	1 lean meat
Stew cubes	1 oz.	1 lean meat
Beans:		
Tempeh	½ cup	2 lean meat 1 starch/bread

▲ EXPANDED FOOD LIST ▲

Medium-Fat Meat

Food value: The following foods contain approximately 7 grams of protein, 5 grams of fat, and 75 calories. Each is one medium-fat meat exchange unless otherwise specified. Most beef and pork roasts or steaks fall into this category.

FOOD	QUANTITY	EXCHANGE
Beef:		
Blade steak or pot roast	1 oz.	1 med. fat meat
Boneless chuck steak or roast, well trimmed	1 oz.	1 med. fat meat
Brisket, lean	1 oz.	1 med. fat meat
Club steak	1 oz.	1 med. fat meat
Corned beef, cured	1 oz.	1 med. fat meat
Ground beef (85% lean)	1 oz.	1 med. fat meat
Ground beef (80% lean)	1 oz.	1 med. fat meat
Ground beef, drained,	½ cup	3 med. fat meat
Meatballs	1 oz.	1 med. fat meat
New York strip steak	1 oz.	1 med. fat meat
Porterhouse steak	1 oz.	1 med. fat meat
Rib roast	1 oz.	1 med. fat meat
Shoulder roast	1 oz.	1 med. fat meat
Sirloin tip roast	1 oz.	1 med. fat meat
T-bone steak	1 oz.	1 med. fat meat
Tongue	1 oz.	1 med. fat meat
Cheese:		
Churny Lite reduced fat Monterey Jack, mild or sharp cheddar, Swiss, American, Colby, Muenster	1 oz.	1 med. fat meat
Dorman's Light part-skim mozzarella, Lo-Chol	1 oz.	1 med. fat meat
Farmers	1 oz.	1 med. fat meat
Heidi Ann natural cheddar style	1 oz.	1 med. fat meat
Kraft flavored spreads jalapeno, olive & pimento, pimiento, pineapple, relish	1 oz.	1 med. fat meat

FOOD	QUANTITY	EXCHANGES
Light Philadelphia cream cheese	1 oz.	1 med. fat meat
Light 'n Lively American, sharp cheddar, Swiss (Kraft)	1 oz.	1 med. fat meat
Mozzarella, natural (part skim)	1 oz.	1 med. fat meat
Parmesan, hard	½ oz.	1 med. fat meat
Parmesan, grated	2 Tbsp.	1 med. fat meat
Ricotta, natural (whole milk)	1 oz.	1 med. fat meat
Romano	½ oz.	1 med. fat meat
Ryser natural cheddar	1 oz.	1 med. fat meat
String cheese	1 oz.	1 med. fat meat
Tendale natural cheddar	1 oz.	1 med. fat meat
Weight Watchers natural cheddar	1 oz.	1 med. fat meat

Eggs:

FOOD	QUANTITY	EXCHANGES
Egg omelet	2 eggs	2 med. fat meat 1 fat

Fish:

FOOD	QUANTITY	EXCHANGES
Anchovy, drained	7	1 med. fat meat
Caviar, black and red, granular	2 Tbsp.	1 med. fat meat
Herring	1 oz.	1 med. fat meat
Mackerel, Atlantic, Pacific & Jack, broiled	1 oz.	1 med. fat meat
Oysters, breaded, fried	3 oz.	1 med. fat meat 1 starch/bread 1 fat
Shrimp, breaded, fried	4 oz. (12 shrimp)	3 med. fat meat 1 starch/bread
Sticks	4	1 med. fat meat 1 starch/bread 1 fat

Lamb:

FOOD	QUANTITY	EXCHANGES
Chops, loin or rib	1 oz.	1 med. fat meat
Leg, roasted	1 oz.	1 med. fat meat
New Zealand, shoulder	1 oz.	1 med. fat meat

Processed Meat:

FOOD	QUANTITY	EXCHANGES
Barbecue loaf, pork, beef	1 oz. (2 slices)	1 med. fat meat
Chicken spread	1 oz. (2 Tbsp.)	1 med. fat meat

FOOD	QUANTITY	EXCHANGES
Ham salad or ham and cheese spread	1 oz. (2 Tbsp.)	1 med. fat meat
Ham and cheese loaf	1 oz.	1 med. fat meat
Headcheese (1 slice)	1 oz.	1 med. fat meat
Liver pate, chicken	1 oz.	1 med. fat meat
Minced ham	1 oz.	1 med. fat meat
Old-fashioned loaf (1 slice)	1 oz.	1 med. fat meat
Turkey cotta salami	1 oz.	1 med. fat meat
Turkey summer sausage	1 oz.	1 med. fat meat
Pork:		
Arm, picnic, roasted or cured	1 oz.	1 med. fat meat
Loin blade	1 oz.	1 med. fat meat
Rump, roasted	1 oz.	1 med. fat meat
Shank, roasted	1 oz.	1 med. fat meat
Shoulder, roasted	1 oz.	1 med. fat meat
Poultry:		
Chicken, dark and light meat with skin	1 oz.	1 med. fat meat
Chicken nuggets	3 oz.	2 med. fat meat 1 starch/bread 1 fat
Chicken patties, breaded, fried	3 oz.	2 med. fat meat 1 starch/bread 1 fat
Southern fried chicken	3 oz.	2 med. fat meat 1 starch/bread 2 fat
Beans:		
Miso	½ cup	1 med. fat meat 2½ starch/bread
Tofu	½ cup (¼ block, 2¼" x 1¾" x 1½")	1 med. fat meat

▲ EXPANDED FOOD LISTS ▲

High-Fat Meat

Food value: The following foods contain approximately 7 grams of protein, 8 grams of fat, and 100 calories. Each is equal to one high-fat meat exchange unless otherwise specified. Prime cuts of meat, meat with a high-fat content, most cheeses, regular luncheon meats or cold cuts, frankfurters, and sausages are in this category.

FOOD	QUANTITY	EXCHANGE
Beef:		
Beef breakfast strips, cured, cooked	2 slices (1 oz.)	1 high fat meat
Barbecue ribs	1 oz.	1 high fat meat
Brisket	1 oz.	1 high fat meat
Corned beef brisket	1 oz.	1 high fat meat
Hamburger, more than 20% fat	1 oz.	1 high fat meat
Ribs	1 oz.	1 high fat meat
Short ribs	1 oz.	1 high fat meat
Prime rib or steaks	1 oz.	1 high fat meat
Cheese:		
Blue	1 oz.	1 high fat meat
Brick	1 oz.	1 high fat meat
Brie	1 oz.	1 high fat meat
Camembert	1 oz.	1 high fat meat
Caraway	1 oz.	1 high fat meat
Cheddar	1 oz.	1 high fat meat
Cheezola, cholesterol free (Fisher)	1 oz.	1 high fat meat
Cheshire	1 oz.	1 high fat meat
Colby	1 oz.	1 high fat meat
Dorman's Light, Swiss, Chedda-Jack, Chedda-Delite, Provolone, Edam	1 oz.	1 high fat meat
Feta	1 oz.	1 high fat meat
Fontina	1 oz.	1 high fat meat
Gjetost	1 oz.	1 high fat meat
Gouda	1 oz.	1 high fat meat
Gruyere	1 oz.	1 high fat meat
Havarti	1 oz.	1 high fat meat

FOOD	QUANTITY	EXCHANGES
Limburger	1 oz.	1 high fat meat
Monterey Jack	1 oz.	1 high fat meat
Mozzarella, whole milk	1 oz.	1 high fat meat
Muenster	1 oz.	1 high fat meat
Neufchatel	1 oz.	1 high fat meat
Pimiento	1 oz.	1 high fat meat
Port du Salut	1 oz.	1 high fat meat
Provolone	1 oz.	1 high fat meat
Ricotta, whole milk	1 oz.	1 high fat meat
Swiss	1 oz.	1 high fat meat
Tilsit	1 oz.	1 high fat meat
Pasteurized Process:		
American or American cheese food	1 oz.	1 high fat meat
Cheese ball or log	1 oz.	1 high fat meat
Cheese spread	2 Tbsp.	1 high fat meat
Cold pack cheese food	1 oz.	1 high fat meat
Pimento	1 oz.	1 high fat meat
Swiss or Swiss cheese food	1 oz.	1 high fat meat
Falafel	3 patties	1 high fat meat
	(2 oz.)	1 starch/bread
		1 fat
Pork:		
Arm picnic	1 oz.	1 high fat meat
Bacon	2 slices	1 high fat meat
Barbecue ribs	1 oz.	1 high fat meat
Breakfast strips, Lean 'n Tasty	2 slices	1 high fat meat
Chitterlings	1 oz.	1 high fat meat
Country ribs	1 oz.	1 high fat meat
Country style ham	1 oz.	1 high fat meat
Pig's feet, cured, pickled	1 oz.	1 high fat meat
Sausage, cooked or 1 patty	2 links	1 high fat meat
Spareribs	1 oz.	1 high fat meat
Poultry:		
Duck	1 oz.	1 high fat meat
Goose	1 oz.	1 high fat meat
Processed Meat:		
Beerwurst	1 oz.	1 high fat meat
Blood sausage (blood pudding)	1 oz.	1 high fat meat
Bologna	1 oz.	1 high fat meat

FOOD	QUANTITY	EXCHANGES
Bratwurst, cooked	1 link	2 high fat meat 1 fat
Braunschweiger	1 link	1 high fat meat
Chorizo	1 link (2 oz.)	2 high fat meat 1 fat
Cocktail wieners	3	1 high fat meat
Frankfurter, beef or beef & pork	1	1 high fat meat 1 fat
Frankfurter, chicken	1	1 high fat meat
Frankfurter, turkey	1	1 high fat meat
Frankfurter, bacon & cheese	1	1 high fat meat 1 fat
Ballpark franks	1	1 high fat meat 2 fat
Kielbase	1 oz.	1 high fat meat
Knockwurst	1 oz.	1 high fat meat
Liver sausage	1 oz.	1 high fat meat
Liverwurst	1 oz.	1 high fat meat
Olive loaf	1 oz.	1 high fat meat
Pastrami	1 oz.	1 high fat meat
Pepperoni	1 oz.	1 high fat meat
Pickle & pimiento loaf	1 oz.	1 high fat meat
Polish sausage	1 oz.	1 high fat meat
Salami	1 oz.	1 high fat meat
Scrapple	1 slice	½ high fat meat ½ starch/bread
Smoked link sausage	1 link	1 high fat meat
Spam	1 oz.	1 high fat meat
Thuringer (summer sausage)	1 oz.	1 high fat meat
Vienna sausage	2	1 high fat meat
Wiener	1	1 high fat meat 1 fat

Nuts—A one-ounce serving of most nuts is counted as 1 high-fat meat plus 1 fat exchange or as 1 medium-fat meat plus 2 fat exchanges. Nuts in very small quantities are counted as fat exchanges. See the fat exchange list for portion sizes.

Nuts:

Almonds	1 oz. (24)	1 med. fat meat 2 fat

FOOD	QUANTITY	EXCHANGES
Cashews	1 oz. (18)	1 med. fat meat 2 fat
Filberts (hazelnuts)	1 oz. (12)	1 med. fat meat 2 fat
Mixed nuts, dry or oil roasted	1 oz. (¼ cup)	1 med. fat meat 2 fat
Peanuts	1 oz. (¼ cup)	1 med. fat meat 2 fat
Pistachios	1 oz. (47)	1 med. fat meat 2 fat
Nut Products:		
Almond butter or almond paste	1 Tbsp.	1 high fat meat **or** 2 fat
Peanut butter, creamy or chunky	1 Tbsp.	1 high fat meat **or** 1 med. fat meat 1 fat
Sesame butter (tahini)	1 Tbsp.	1 high fat meat
Seeds:		
Pumpkin or squash	1 oz. (142)	1 med. fat meat 2 fat
Sunflower	1 oz. (¼ cup)	1 med. fat meat 2 fat
Watermelon	1 oz. (95)	1 med. fat meat 2 fat

▲ GUIDELINES ▲

Cheese

Cheese is a nutritious food, providing protein, calcium, vitamin A, and other nutrients. However, cheese often provides more fat than an equal portion of meat. Traditional cheeses usually contain eight or more grams of fat per ounce, predominantly saturated fat. In addition, cheese also contains cholesterol. How much fat and cholesterol a cheese contains depends on the type of milk used in its production. Milk used may be extra rich, whole, 2 percent or skim and may also have butterfat (milkfat) added.

The curds (milk solids) are pressed into "natural" cheese, while the whey (milk liquid) is either discarded or recycled to make mysost, primost, ricotta, or other whey-based cheeses. It may also be used for cottage cheese or cream cheese. Processed cheeses are a blend of natural cheeses, usually the high fat cheddar, Colby or Swiss.

Cheese is also a relatively high sodium food, containing about 150 to 200 milligrams of sodium per ounce. Processed cheeses contain twice as much sodium (350 milligrams per ounce).

The fat content of cheese, if listed on the label, is indicated in one of two ways: grams of fat per ounce or by percent of fat. The percent of fat is equal to the grams of fat per 100 grams (3½ ounces) of cheese. Unfortunately, there is no easy rule of thumb for distinguishing low-fat from high-fat cheese without reading the label or food composition table. Low-fat or high-fat cheeses can be soft or hard, white or yellow. Fortunately, modern technology and growing consumer interest have stimulated cheesemakers to produce greater varieties of low-fat cheeses with flavor and texture similar to that of traditional higher fat cheeses.

An average serving of cheese is usually one ounce. This is typically one average slice (prewrapped cheese slices may be only ¾ ounce) or 1¼-inch cube. Low-fat cheeses can usually be substituted for higher fat cheeses in recipes without much difficulty.

The following guidelines can help you decide which cheeses to select. They are based on the grams of fat per ounce of cheese.

▲ Cheese with 1 to 3 grams of fat per ounce:
These cheeses are made primarily from skim milk and are included on the lean meat list.

▲ Cheese with 4 to 5 grams of fat per ounce:
The fat, saturated fat and cholesterol content of these cheeses is similar to 1 ounce of medium fat meat.

▲ Cheese with 6 to 8 grams of fat per ounce:
These cheeses are made from whole milk and contain a large amount of saturated fat and cholesterol. They are included on the high-fat meat exchange list. Total fat is more than a teaspoon per ounce of cheese.

▲   Cheese with 6 to 8 grams of low cholesterol fat per ounce (filled skim milk cheese):
Though similar in total fat to regular cheese, filled cheese is low in cholesterol and saturated fat. However, it is still included on the high fat meat list because of the total fat content. Select filled cheeses made with corn, cottonseed, safflower, or sunflower seed oils. Avoid coconut or palm oils.

▲   Cheese with 9 to 11 grams of fat per ounce:
These cheeses are made from whole milk with added butterfat (milkfat). They are high-fat cheeses that contain up to one tablespoon of fat per ounce. One ounce of these cheeses is one high-fat meat exchange plus one fat exchange.

Word List

Natural cheeses:	These are made from curdled milk through different types of processing. They may or may not be aged or ripened to make different types of cheese.
Processed cheeses:	American, cheese food or cheese spreads are a blend of one or more natural cheeses that are ground, blended, or heated together. This process provides uniformity of product and increases the shelf life.
Cheese foods:	At least 51 percent of the product is pasteurized processed cheese, with cream, milk, skim milk, or whey added.
Cheese spreads:	These are cheese foods with an edible stabilizer and extra moisture added to allow smooth spreading at room temperature.

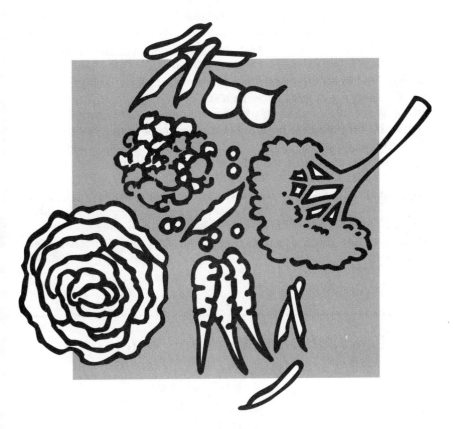

VEGETABLE EXCHANGES

Linked with fruits on the second layer of the Food Guide Pyramid are all the wonderful vegetable choices. Because vegetables are great for you, choose 3 to 5 servings per day. Vegetables grow in abundant variety—from A (asparagus) to Z (zucchini). They are generally low in calories and carbohydrate but excellent sources of fiber and important vitamins and minerals. Most dark-green and deep-yellow vegetables excel as a source of vitamin A. Many dark-green vegetables also supply valuable amounts of vitamin C. Meals would be very drab without the color, crispness, tang, texture, and flavor of vegetables.

One pound of raw vegetables usually yields four half-cup cooked portions. Cooking greens, such as kale and spinach, are the exception: one pound yields 8 to 12 half-cup servings, cooked.

One half-cup serving of many cooked vegetables is one vegetable exchange. When eaten raw, in amounts less than one cup, vegetables have less than 20 calories and therefore may be considered free food.

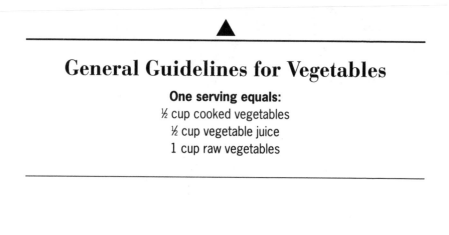

General Guidelines for Vegetables

One serving equals:
½ cup cooked vegetables
½ cup vegetable juice
1 cup raw vegetables

▲ EXPANDED FOOD LIST ▲

Vegetable

Food value: The following foods contain about 5 grams of carbohydrate, 2 grams of protein, and 25 calories. They also contain 2 to 3 grams of fiber. Each equals one vegetable exchange.

FOOD	QUANTITY	EXCHANGES
Amaranth, cooked	½ cup	1 vegetable
Artichoke, French/globe, cooked base and soft end of leaves	½ medium	1 vegetable
Artichoke heart, cooked	½ heart	1 vegetable
Asparagus	7 spears	1 vegetable
Bamboo shoots, cooked	½ cup	1 vegetable
Beans, snap, cooked	½ cup	1 vegetable
Bell pepper	1 medium	1 vegetable
Beets, cooked	½ cup	1 vegetable
Bok choy, Chinese chard,	1 cup	1 vegetable
White mustard cabbage, cooked	½ cup	1 vegetable
Borscht	½ cup	1 vegetable
Broccoli, cooked	1 medium stalk **or** ½ cup	1 vegetable
Brussels sprouts	3 sprouts	1 vegetable
Cabbage, boiled	½ cup	1 vegetable
Cactus leaves, Napoles	1 medium leaf	1 vegetable
Carrots	1 large **or** 2 small	1 vegetable
Carrot juice	¼ cup	1 vegetable
Cauliflower	⅙ medium head	1 vegetable
Celery	2 medium stalks	1 vegetable
Chayote, cooked	½ cup **or** ½ medium squash	1 vegetable
Chinese cabbage, Nappa, raw	2 cups shredded	1 vegetable
Collards, boiled	½ cup	1 vegetable
Cucumber	⅓ medium	1 vegetable
Daikon, raw	1 cup	1 vegetable
Dandelion greens, cooked	½ cup	1 vegetable

FOOD	QUANTITY	EXCHANGES
Dips:		
Jalapeno bean	2 tablespoons	1 vegetable
Salsa	¼ cup	1 vegetable
Taco	¼ cup	1 vegetable
Eggplant, cooked	¾ cup 1" cubes	1 vegetable
Jerusalem artichokes	¼ cup	1 vegetable
Jicama, raw	½ cup	1 vegetable
Kale, cooked	½ cup	1 vegetable
Kohlrabi, raw or cooked	½ cup	1 vegetable
Leeks, raw	⅓ cup chopped	1 vegetable
Lettuce, iceberg	⅙ large head	1 vegetable
Lettuce, leaf	3 cups shredded	1 vegetable
Mushrooms	8	1 vegetable
Mustard greens, cooked	1 cup	1 vegetable
Okra, cooked	8 average pods **or** ½ cup sliced	1 vegetable
Onions, cooked	½ cup	1 vegetable
Pea pods, Chinese pea pods, snow peas, cooked	½ cup	1 vegetable
Pumpkin, mashed	½ cup	1 vegetable
Rhubarb	1 cup	1 vegetable
Rutabaga, cooked	½ cup	1 vegetable
Sauerkraut, canned	½ cup	1 vegetable
Sprouts, alfalfa, bean, soybean	1 cup raw **or** ¾ cup cooked	1 vegetable
Summer squash, cooked	½ cup slices	1 vegetable
Tomatillos	2	1 vegetable
Tomatoes, red, raw	1	1 vegetable
Tomatoes, stewed	½ cup	1 vegetable
Tomato juice	½ cup	1 vegetable
Tomato paste	2 Tbsp.	1 vegetable
Tomato puree	¼ cup	1 vegetable
Tomato sauce	⅓ cup	1 vegetable
Turnips, mashed	½ cup	1 vegetable
Turnip greens, cooked	½ cup	1 vegetable
Vegetable juice cocktail	½ cup	1 vegetable
Water chestnuts, Chinese, canned	½ cup slices	1 vegetable
Yardlong beans, cooked	4 pods	1 vegetable

Word List

Artichoke: Globe artichokes are large, unopened buds from a thistle-like plant. You eat them by pulling off the leaves one by one from the cooked artichoke and drawing them between your teeth. The tender heart can be eaten whole. The fuzzy choke at the center should be cut or scooped out and discarded.

Artichoke, Jerusalem (sun choke): North American native tuber from the sunflower plant. Has a sweet, nutty flavor and can be served raw or boiled and used as a potato substitute.

Bean sprouts: Tender shoots of the soya, mung or curd bean. They may be eaten raw or cooked.

Bok choy: Also known as Chinese chard or white mustard cabbage. It is a green, leafy Oriental vegetable with slender white stems. It resembles both Swiss chard and celery. Bok choy is a sweet, mild-tasting vegetable that can be stir-fried or served raw.

Cactus leaves (Napoles): A green, crisp and tender Mexican vegetable with a flavor and texture similar to green beans. To prepare, remove the "eyes" which contain the cactus thorns with a sharp knife; cut leaf into cubes and cook in water for 10 minutes.

Chayote: A squash-like vegetable that is light green and pear-shaped. It can be used in any recipe that calls for winter or summer squash.

Chinese cabbage (Nappa): A member of the cabbage family, it has a long slender head with long, pale green and white wrinkled leaves. It has a tender texture and a mild, delicate flavor.

Daikon: A large white radish that can be served raw or pickled. The flavor is slightly hotter than an ordinary radish.

Eggplant: A dark purple, glossy and pear-shaped vegetable which originated in the Orient.

Greens (cooking): Mild flavored greens include beet tops, dandelion, spinach, and collards. Strong-flavored greens include kale, mustard, Swiss chard, and turnip tops.

Jicama: A large, lumpy tuber with dull brown skin. The inside is white, crisp, and juicy with a water chestnut flavor. Delicious eaten raw.

Kohlrabi: A member of the cabbage family. Bulbs may be steamed or eaten raw and have a delicate turnip-like taste.

Leeks: They resemble green onions in shape and flavor but are much larger and milder.

Okra: Slim, tapered pods that are sometimes nicknamed "lady's fingers." Okra can be used as a thickening agent in soups or stews.

Snow peas: These are sometimes called sugar peas or Chinese peas and have transparent green pods.

Summer squash: They have soft shells and include yellow crookneck, straightneck, zucchini (Italian squash), pattypans (scallop or button), and spaghetti squash.

Yellow Crookneck: They have a warted, light yellow skin with a creamy yellow flesh and are curved at the neck.

Pattypans: They are disc-shaped with a ribbed edge, giving them a scalloped appearance. The skin is pale green when young, white when older. The entire squash can be eaten.

Spaghetti: An edible gourd that is light green in color with a smooth skin.

Straightneck: They are similar to the crookneck but relatively straight.

Zucchini: Straight in shape with a skin color that is dark green.

Tomatillos: Commonly known as ground tomatoes, they are small, round, firm-textured, husk-covered green vegetables. When eaten raw they have a tart taste.

Water chestnuts: They are brown on the outside and have a white inside with a nutlike flavor. They remain crisp even after cooking and are commonly used in Chinese cookery.

Winter squash: They have hard, firm shells and include acorn, buttercup, banana, Hubbard, and Mediterranean squash. Winter squash is higher in calories than summer squash; a one-cup cooked portion is included on the starch/bread list.

Acorn: It is acorn-shaped with yellowish, sweet tasting flesh. It is usually cooked unpeeled because of its tough skin.

Banana: It is cylindrical in shape and has a pale olive gray color that changes to creamy pink in storage. It is usually sold by the piece.

Buttercup: Drum-shaped with a turban cap at the blossom end, it has green skin and bright yellow-orange flesh.

Butternut: Cylindrical in shape with a bulbous base, it has dark yellow skin and yellow orange flesh.

Hubbard: Heavy for its size, it has a bright yellow-orange flesh and is usually sold by the piece.

Mediterranean: A long cylindrical shape and slightly bulbous at one end, it is beige in color with a ridged skin and bright orange interior. Also sold by the piece.

Yardlong beans: Long and slender, yard-long beans are related to black-eyed peas in appearance, taste, and texture. They are perfect in long-cooked dishes, adding a chewy-firm, almost meaty texture and taste.

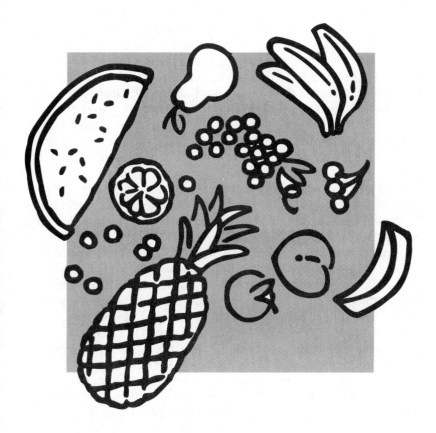

FRUIT EXCHANGES

Fruits—fresh, dried, canned or frozen without added sugar—are also on the second layer of the Food Guide Pyramid and are excellent choices. They provide important amounts of vitamin A and C and potassium. They are low in fat and sodium. The Food Guide Pyramid suggests two to four servings of fruits a day.

If in doubt about portion sizes, a good rule of thumb is ½ cup of fresh or canned fruit or juice, ¼ cup of dried fruit, or the equivalent of one small- to medium-sized fresh fruit. Fruits vary in portion size because of their water content. Fruits with a higher water content (for example, strawberries and watermelon) have a larger portion size than fruits with a low water content (for example, bananas and dried fruits). If you are unsure of the correct portion for dried or canned fruits, use the same amount you would for fresh fruit. The difference in the fruit is simply the water content. The portion sizes for dried fruit seem small compared to fresh fruit, but the amount of calories and carbohydrate is the same.

Canned fruit may be packed in fruit juice or its own juice, water-packed, or artificially sweetened. The serving size for fruit packed in juice includes a small amount of juice. If you wish to use more juice, use a smaller serving of fruit. Instead of one-half cup use one-third cup fruit with juice for your portion size. Liquid from water-packed fruit need not be counted. Pass up fruit canned in heavy syrups.

Choose 100 percent fruit juices. If fruit juices or fruits contain sugar, this must be stated on the label. If no mention is made of sugar, you can assume the fruit or juice does not contain sugar. Fruit "drinks," "ades," or "punches" contain only a little juice and lots of added sugars. They are not as good a choice as fruit juices.

▲

General Guidelines for Fruits

One serving equals:
1 small to medium fresh fruit
½ cup canned
¼ cup dried
⅓ to ½ cup fruit juice

▲ EXPANDED FOOD LIST ▲

Fruit

Food value: The following foods contain approximately 15 grams of carbohydrate and 60 calories. Fresh, frozen, and dried fruits have about 2 grams of fiber per serving. Fruit juices have very little fiber. Each of the following is one fruit exchange.

FOOD	QUANTITY	EXCHANGES
Apples:		
Sliced, raw	½ cup	1 fruit
Dehydrated, dried	¼ cup	1 fruit
Apricots:		
Raw	3 medium	1 fruit
Canned, juice pack	4 halves	1 fruit
Dried	7 halves	1 fruit
Berries:		
Blackberries, raw	¾ cup	1 fruit
Blueberries, raw	⅓ cup	1 fruit
Boysenberries, frozen, unsweetened	1 cup	1 fruit
Elderberries, raw	½ cup	1 fruit
Gooseberries	1 cup	1 fruit

FOOD	QUANTITY	EXCHANGES
Loganberries	¾ cup	1 fruit
Mulberries	1 cup	1 fruit
Raspberries, raw	1 cup	1 fruit
Strawberries, frozen, unsweetened	1 cup	1 fruit
Wild blueberries	½ cup	1 fruit
Breadfruit, raw	⅛ medium	1 fruit
Carambala (star fruit)	1½ fruit	1 fruit
Cherimoya, raw	½	1 fruit
Cherries:		
Sour red, canned light syrup pack	⅓ cup	1 fruit
Sweet, raw	12	1 fruit
Sweet, canned, juice pack	½ cup	1 fruit
Crabapples, raw	¾ cup	1 fruit
Cranberry-orange relish	2 Tbsp.	1 fruit
Cranberry sauce, canned	2 Tbsp.	1 fruit
Currants, red and white, raw	1 cup	1 fruit
Feijoa	3 fruit **or**	1 fruit
	½ cup puree	
Fruit bars	1 (½ oz.)	1 fruit
Fruit cocktail, canned, juice pack	½ cup	1 fruit
Fruit roll-ups	1 (½ oz.)	1 fruit
Fruit salad, canned, juice pack	½ cup	1 fruit
Granadilla, passion fruit, raw	3	1 fruit
Grapefruit sections	¾ cup	1 fruit
Ground-cherries, raw	1 cup	1 fruit
Guavas	1 fruit	1 fruit
Homli fruit	1 fruit	1 fruit
Kiwifruit	1½ medium **or**	1 fruit
	1 large	
Kumquats, raw	5	1 fruit
Lemon	3 medium	1 fruit
Lime	3 medium	1 fruit
Loquats, raw	12	1 fruit
Lychees, litchis	½ cup **or** 10	1 fruit
Mangoes, raw	½ fruit	1 fruit
Melons:		
Cantaloupe, raw	1 cup cubed	1 fruit
Casaba, raw	1½ cup cubed	1 fruit
Honeydew, raw	1 cup cubed	1 fruit

FOOD	QUANTITY	EXCHANGES
Melon balls, frozen	1 cup	1 fruit
Nectarines, raw	1	1 fruit
Papayas, raw	½ fruit	1 fruit
Peaches, raw	¾ cup slices	1 fruit
canned, juice pack	2 halves **or** ½ cup slices	1 fruit
Pears, raw	¾ cup slices	1 fruit
canned, juice pack	2 halves	1 fruit
Pears, Asian, raw	1 fruit	1 fruit
Persimmons, raw	½ fruit	1 fruit
Pineapple, canned, juice pack	1½ slices	1 fruit
Plantains, cooked	⅓ cup slices	1 fruit
Plums, canned, juice pack	3 fruits	1 fruit
Pomegranates, raw	½ fruit	1 fruit
Prickly pears, raw	1½ fruit	1 fruit
Pomelo, raw	¾ cup sections	1 fruit
Quince, raw	1	1 fruit
Rhubarb, diced	2 cups	1 fruit
Sapota, raw	1 small	1 fruit
Spreadable fruit		
Kraft reduced calorie	8 tsp.	1 fruit
Poiret fruit spread	1 Tbsp.	1 fruit
Polaner all fruit	4 tsp.	1 fruit
Smucker's light	8 tsp.	1 fruit
Smucker's low sugar	8 tsp.	1 fruit
Smucker's simply fruit	4 tsp.	1 fruit
Welch totally fruit	4 tsp.	1 fruit
Tamarinds, raw	12	1 fruit
Tangelos	1	1 fruit
Tangerines, canned, juice pack	⅔ cup	1 fruit
Ugli fruit	¾ cup	1 fruit
Juices:		
Apple juice	½ cup	1 fruit
Apricot nectar	⅓ cup	1 fruit
Beef broth & tomato juice	5.5 fl. oz. can	1 fruit
Catawba juice	¾ cup	1 fruit
Clam & tomato juice	5.5 fl. oz. can	1 fruit
Cranberry juice cocktail	½ cup	1 fruit
Cranapple juice drink	⅓ cup	1 fruit

FOOD	QUANTITY	EXCHANGES
Low calorie cranberry or cranapple or cranraspberry juice cocktail	1 cup	1 fruit
Gatorade	1 cup	1 fruit
Grape juice	½ cup	1 fruit
Hawaiian Punch, low calorie	1 cup	1 fruit
Lemon juice	1 cup	1 fruit
Lime juice	1 cup	1 fruit
New Breakfast juice	½ cup	1 fruit
Orange-grapefruit juice	½ cup	1 fruit
Papaya nectar	⅓ cup	1 fruit
Passion-fruit juice	½ cup	1 fruit
Peach nectar	½ cup	1 fruit
Pear nectar	⅓ cup	1 fruit
Pineapple juice	⅓ cup	1 fruit
Prune juice	⅓ cup	1 fruit
Tangerine juice	½ cup	1 fruit
Tomato juice	1½ cup	1 fruit
V-8 vegetable cocktail	1½ cup	1 fruit

Word List

Breadfruit: Starchy and melon-shaped, it is used as a vegetable in Caribbean and Latin American cookery. It is boiled or baked like a potato and has a taste similar to bread, which is how it gets its name.

Carambola (star fruit): When this fruit is cut crosswise, it has a star shape. It has a golden yellow color with juicy flesh and crisp texture.

Cherimoya: A heart-shaped fruit that is green when ripe and has a skin marked with petal-like indentations. When ripened and chilled, the flesh has a sherbet-like texture. It is also called sweet sop, sherbet fruit, or custard apple.

Feijoa: It looks like an elongated guava and has an aromatic pulp that combines the taste of pineapple, quince, spruce, and Concord grapes with a menthol-lemon tang. The inside is eaten fresh or used as an ingredient in fruit salads and jams.

Granadilla (passion fruit): It has the size and shape of an egg, a tough purple skin, and yellow flesh with black seeds and appears shriveled when ripe and ready to eat. It reminded early South American missionaries of Christ's crown of thorns, so they named it "passion fruit."

Guava: A sweet, juicy fruit whose skin ranges in color from green to yellow with an inside that can be white, deep pink, or salmon red. It has many small seeds in the center and is native to Mexico and South America.

Homli fruit: A cross between a grapefruit and an orange. It has a greenish skin with orange flesh. The fruit is slightly sweeter than a grapefruit but not as sweet as an orange.

Kiwifruit: Brown and elongated with a fuzzy skin, the inside is lime green and similar in texture to the American gooseberry. It is also known as a "Chinese gooseberry" because of its Chinese origin. It now comes from New Zealand or California.

Kumquat: A small, orange fruit of Chinese origin. It has a very definite citrus flavor. The skin is sweet and the flesh has a tangy flavor. The seeds should be removed before eating.

Loquat: A small, round fruit with yellow-orange skin and pale yellow to orange flesh with black seeds. The flavor is somewhat like a blend of banana and pineapple. It comes from a tropical, ornamental evergreen tree, is very juicy, not too sweet, and best when eaten very ripe.

Lychee (litchi): An ancient Chinese fruit that is like a strawberry in shape and size. It has a reddish brown, hard skin that is easy to peel. The flesh is white and mild flavored with a single seed and has the consistency of a fresh grape.

Mango: Mangoes may vary in size and shape, depending on the variety and area in which they are grown. They are generally large and oval-shaped with a tough skin that can be green, yellow, red, or a combination of the three, with more reds and yellows as the fruit ripens. Their flesh is orange-yellow, has a spicy aroma, and a rich flavor that is a blend of apricot and pineapple. They must be fully ripe before eating.

Melons:

Cantaloupe (Muskmelon):	A melon with a cream-colored netting over golden under-color, orange flesh color, and a distinctive-sweet flavor, musky-sweet aroma.
Casaba:	Large round melon with deeply furrowed, yellow rind and a creamy white flesh. Tastes similar to honeydew, little aroma.
Honeydew:	Waxy skin, white and green outside, inside has a cream to pale green flesh and a juicy, sweet, honey aroma.
Orange honeydew:	Shaped like a honeydew, it has a soft orange color to its skin with a salmon-colored flesh.
Golden honeydew:	Golden tinge to its skin, orange-like colored flesh, juicy and similar to a cantaloupe.
Pink honeydew:	Pink tinge to its skin, pinkish flesh, juicy. Tastes sweet and has a honey-like aroma.
Papaya:	It is really a very large berry with a deep green outer peel and yellow-to-orange inside. It has a mild flavor and contains an enzyme, papain, that is extracted and sold as a tenderizer. It can be eaten fresh or cooked.
Pear, Asian:	Originally from China, it looks like a very small pear. Crisp and russeted, it is also known as apple-pear, Japanese pear, pear-apples, and Chalea.
Persimmon:	It is bright orange in color and has a smooth shiny skin that is removed before eating. It is known as the "apple of the Orient." Persimmons must be very soft before eating or they have a very sour, astringent taste.
Plantain:	A "cooking banana" with greenish, rough skin. It is an important staple food in tropical countries. Used as a vegetable, the fruit is starchy and is never eaten raw. It can be baked, boiled, or prepared in much the same way as potatoes.
Pomegranate:	The name means "apple with many seeds." It is about the size of an orange with a hard skin and deep red color. The inside is filled with edible sweet seeds which are the only edible part of the fruit; the pulp is too bitter.
Prickly pears:	The fruit of a species of cactus; also called cactus pear,

Indian fig, and Barberry fig. It has a yellow to crimson skin that is covered with spines. The inside is purple-red to yellow and has a sweet taste similar to watermelon.

Pomelo: This citrus fruit, the tropical ancestor of the grapefruit, has a thick rind and sweet, red pulp. The flavor is mild rather than bitter.

Quince: A very ancient fruit that has hard, tart meat that is not good for eating. Quince is best when made into a sauce or baked.

Sapota: It resembles a green apple in appearance; fruit should be firm with greenish to yellow-green color. It has a custard-like consistency and flavor that some believe tastes like vanilla ice cream. Also called custard apple, it can be eaten fresh.

Tamarind: A cinnamon-brown, long, flattened pod used in Oriental chutneys and curries.

Tangelo: A citrus fruit with loose skin that is a hybrid of the tangerine. It is the size of a large orange, but the flavor is slightly more tart.

Ugli fruit: Native to Jamaica, it is about the size of a grapefruit with a disfigured, rough peel. The skin peels off like a tangerine and the pulp is very juicy with an orange-like flavor.

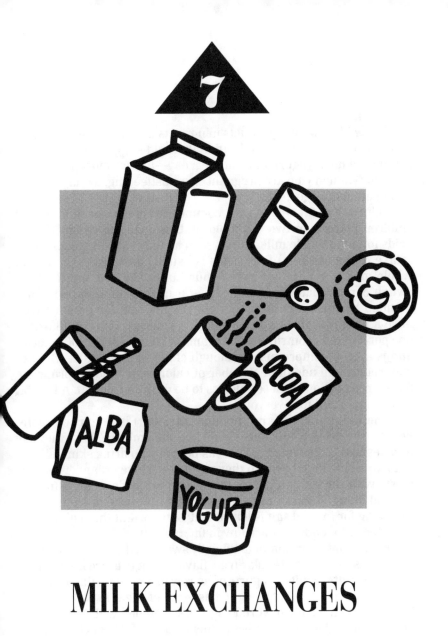

MILK EXCHANGES

Milk and milk products join meats and meat substitutes as good food choices. The Food Guide Pyramid suggests two to three servings of milk, yogurt, and cheese a day—two for most people and three for women who are pregnant or breastfeeding, teenagers, and young adults to age 24.

Skim or low-fat milk is the recommended choice, beginning with children more than two years old. Babies need the essential fatty acids found in whole milk, but as soon as they eat solid foods, their intake of the essential fatty acids is usually adequate. The use of whole milk is generally recommended until age two and then the switch can be made to skim or low-fat milk. Skim milk is recommended because it contains little or no fat, and for persons who have a weight problem, it is also low in calories. One cup (8 oz.) of one percent milk contributes 2.5 grams of fat and about 100 calories and is a good compromise. Although children and adults who are lean require an adequate number of calories, it is not appropriate for a large portion of these calories to be derived from fat. A low-fat diet is important for everyone.

The liking for fat (and, incidentally, salt) is a learned taste. People who drink whole milk do not like skim milk because they say it tastes like "blue water." Whereas people who drink skim milk do not like whole milk because they say it tastes like cream. This contrasts with the human desire for sweetness, which seems to be a natural liking. Babies naturally like the sweet taste of fruits. Since the liking for fat and salt is learned, it is important that children be introduced to foods that are low in fat and salt.

Plain, nonfat, or nonfat artificially sweetened yogurts are excellent milk substitutes. Regular fruit-flavored yogurts are not an ideal milk substitute. Fruited yogurts often rely on imitation flavoring and coloring and contain six to eight teaspoons of sugar in eight ounces. You can buy the fruit-flavored yogurts sweetened with NutraSweet or other noncaloric sweeteners or buy plain nonfat yogurt and flavor it yourself with fresh or unsweetened fruit or fruit juices. If desired, add a noncaloric sweetener like Equal for additional sweetness.

▲
_____

General Guidelines for Milk

One serving equals:
1 cup skim or 1% milk
8 ounces plain nonfat yogurt
6 to 8 ounces artificially sweetened fruit
flavored nonfat yogurts

_____

▲ EXPANDED FOOD LIST ▲

Milk

Food Value: The following foods contain approximately 12 grams of carbohydrate, 8 grams of protein, a trace of fat, and 90 calories, similar to one cup of skim milk. The amount of fat in milk is measured in percent of butterfat. The calories vary, depending on the type of milk and its butterfat content. An 8-ounce glass of 2 percent milk contains 5 grams of fat and 120 calories. A glass of whole milk (3 to 4 percent) has 8 grams of fat and 150 calories.

FOOD	QUANTITY	EXCHANGES
Alba cocoa mix, powder	~19 g packet	1 skim milk
Alba Fit 'n Frosty	~21 g packet	1 skim milk
Buttermilk, cultured	1 cup	1 skim milk
Chocolate milk, 1% milk	8 fl. oz.	1 skim milk
		1 starch/bread
Cocoa/hot chocolate, sweetened with aspartame	~.5 oz. packet or ¾ heaping teaspoon in 6 fl. oz. water	½ skim milk
Cocoa mix, 50 calorie mix	6 oz. prepared	½ skim milk
Custard	½ cup	1 skim milk
		1½ fat

FOOD	QUANTITY	EXCHANGES
Custard style yogurt, plain	8 oz.	1½ skim milk 1 fat
Custard style yogurt, flavored	6 oz.	1 skim milk 1 fruit, 1 fat
Eggnog, nonalcoholic	8 fl. oz.	1 skim milk 1½ starch/bread 3 fat
Evaporated skim milk, canned	½ cup	1 skim milk
Filled milk	1 cup	1 skim milk 1 fat
Goat milk	1 cup	1 skim milk 1½ fat
Instant Breakfast, all flavors	1 pkg. dry mix only	1 skim milk 1 fruit
Instant Breakfast, all varieties	1 pkg. & 8 oz. skim milk	2 skim milk 1 fruit
Instant Breakfast, diet all varieties	1 pkg. dry mix only	1 skim milk
Instant Breakfast, diet all varieties	1 pkg. & 8 oz. skim milk	2 skim milk
Lactaid	1 cup	1 skim milk
Skim milk, dry	¼ cup	1 skim milk
Soy milk	1 cup	½ skim milk 1 fat
Weight Watchers shake mixes, all varieties	1 envelope	1 skim milk
Yogurt, fruit flavored, sweetened with aspartame	6 to 8 oz.	1 skim milk
Yogurt lite, all varieties	6 oz.	1 skim milk
Yogurt, nonfat, vanilla	8 oz.	1½ skim milk 1 fruit

Word List

Filled: Milk that contains fats or oils other than milk fat.

Lactaid: Lactose, which is milk sugar, is reduced, usually to 3 grams per cup. Often useful for persons with a lactose intolerance.

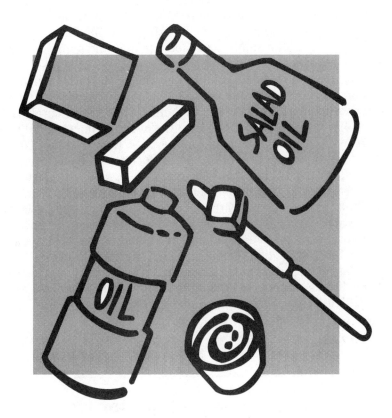

FAT EXCHANGES

Squeezed into the tip of the Food Guide Pyramid are the foods to be careful of—fats and sugars. These foods supply calories, but little or no vitamins and minerals. By using these foods sparingly, you can have a diet that supplies needed vitamins and minerals without excess calories.

It is recommended the amount of fat in the diet be limited to about 30 percent or less of our calories each day. For persons eating approximately 1,500 calories a day, this is about 50 grams of fat, and for 2,400 calories, 80 grams of fat. The average American fat intake is 37 to 45 percent of the total calories or 65 to 105 grams of fat.

It is the saturated fat in the diet, associated with elevating blood cholesterol levels, that should be reduced, however. Saturated fats, usually of animal origin, are solid at room temperature. Unsaturated fats, either monounsaturated or polyunsaturated, should be used in place of saturated fats whenever possible. Unsaturated fats are primarily of vegetable origin and are liquid at room temperature. These fats are thought to help reduce cholesterol levels.

Nuts and seeds in small amounts are counted as fat exchanges, but in larger amounts as 1 medium-fat meat and 2 fat exchanges or as 1 high-fat meat exchange and 1 fat exchange. See the high-fat meat exchange list for portion sizes.

▲

General Guidelines for Fats

One serving equals:
1 teaspoon margarine or butter
1 tablespoon reduced-calorie margarine
1 teaspoon mayonnaise or oil
1 tablespoon regular salad dressing
2 tablespoons low-calorie salad dressing
2 tablespoons sour cream

▲ EXPANDED FOOD LIST ▲

Fat

Food value: The following foods contain approximately 5 grams of fat and 45 calories. They are each equivalent to one fat exchange.

FOOD	QUANTITY	EXCHANGES
Unsaturated Fats:		
Avocado	⅛ or	1 fat
	2 Tbsp. mashed	
Blue cheese salad dressing	2 teaspoons	1 fat
Low-calorie salad dressings	2 tablespoons	1 fat
French, Italian, Russian,		
Thousand Island		
Margarines:		
Diet	1 tablespoon	1 fat
Liquid	1 teaspoon	1 fat
Reduced-calorie	1 tablespoon	1 fat
Tub	1 teaspoon	1 fat
Whipped	2 teaspoons	1 fat
Mayonnaise-type	2 teaspoons	1 fat
Mayonnaise-type, Light	1 tablespoon	1 fat
Nuts, chopped	1 tablespoon	1 fat
Nuts:		
Almonds	7	1 fat
Brazil nuts	2 medium	1 fat
Cashews	5 medium	1 fat
Filberts (hazelnuts)	5	1 fat
Macadamia	3	1 fat
Mixed	5 to 6	1 fat
Peanuts	⅓ oz.	1 fat
Pecans	5 halves	1 fat
Pine nuts, pignolia	1 tablespoon	1 fat
	(25)	
Pistachios	15	1 fat
Walnuts	4 halves or	1 fat
	1 Tbsp. chopped	

FOOD	QUANTITY	EXCHANGES
Peanut butter	1 teaspoon	1 fat
Regular salad dressings	1 tablespoon	1 fat
Sandwich spread	2 teaspoons	1 fat
Seeds:		
Pumpkin and squash	45	1 fat
Sesame seeds	1 tablespoon	1 fat
Soybean	50	1 fat
Sunflower seed kernels	1 tablespoon	1 fat
Sesame butter (tahini)	½ tablespoon	1 fat
Tartar sauce	2 teaspoons	1 fat
Thousand island or Russian dressing	2 teaspoons	1 fat
Vegetable oils	1 teaspoon	1 fat
Vinegar & oil dressing	2 teaspoons	1 fat
Saturated Fats:		
Anchiote, prepared	1 teaspoon	1 fat
Cheese sauce	2 tablespoon	1 fat
Cheese spread	1 tablespoon	1 fat
Chicken fat	1 teaspoon	1 fat
Chicken liver pate	2 tablespoons	1 fat
Chitterlings, fried	2 tablespoons	1 fat
Coconut	2 tablespoons	1 fat
Cream cheese	1 tablespoon	1 fat
Cream cheese, light	5 teaspoons	1 fat
Cream cheese dip	1 tablespoon	1 fat
Creamers:		
Liquid	1 Tbsp. (1 oz.)	1 fat
Powdered	4 teaspoons	1 fat
Dips, sour-cream based	2 tablespoons	1 fat
Dips, light	¼ cup	1 fat
Gravy:		
Canned	¼ cup	1 fat
From mix	½ cup	1 fat
Half and half cream	2 tablespoons	1 fat
Lard	1 teaspoon	1 fat
Neufchatel	¾ oz.	1 fat
Shortenings	1 teaspoon	1 fat
Sour cream	2 tablespoons	1 fat
Sour cream, lean or light	3 tablespoons	1 fat

FOOD	QUANTITY	EXCHANGES
Whipped butter	2 teaspoons	1 fat
Whipped toppings:		
From mix	5 tablespoons	1 fat
Frozen	3 tablespoons	1 fat

Word List

Macadamia nut: Nut from the tall evergreen silk-oak tree; hard-shelled, shiny round nut with delicate flavor. Grown in Hawaii.

Pine nut: Edible sweet flavored nut produced in the pine cone of the nut-bearing pine tree; looks like a large grain of rice. Also called pinon or pignolia.

Pistachio nut: Seed of a red fruit that has a double shell. The natural color of the seed is green.

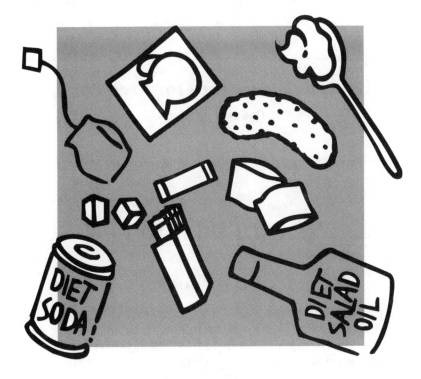

FREE FOODS

Free foods are those with relatively few calories, fewer than 20 per serving. Limit free foods to a total of 50 to 60 calories per day or a total of two to three servings, divided between meals and snacks.

General Guidelines for Free Foods

One serving equals:
20 calories or less per serving

▲ EXPANDED FOOD LIST ▲

Free Foods

Food value: The following foods are noncaloric or negligible in calories (fewer than 20 calories per serving). Maximum serving size is noted when the amount needs to be limited; larger serving sizes contain more than 20 calories. Only one serving of these foods should be eaten at a meal or snack.

FOOD	QUANTITY	EXCHANGES
A-1 sauce or steak sauce	1 tablespoon	Free
Bacos	1 teaspoon	Free
Beverage or drink mixes		
Kool-Aid, powder only		Free
Sugar Free		Free
Sugar free teas		Free
Sugar free iced tea mix		Free

FOOD	QUANTITY	EXCHANGES
Tang sugar free breakfast beverage crystals		Free
Bran, unprocessed	2 tablespoons	Free
Brewer's yeast	2 teaspoons	Free
Butter Buds, dry	3 teaspoons	Free
Candies:		
Gummy bears, dietetic	2	Free
Hard candy, dietetic or sugar free	1 piece	Free
Chewing gum:		
Bubble, sugarless	1 piece	Free
Sugarless	2 pieces	Free
Club soda (not tonic or quinine water)	1	Free
Cocktail sauce	1 tablespoon	Free
Cocoa, dry powder	1 tablespoon	Free
Coffee whiteners:		
Coffee-Mate, liquid	1 tablespoon	Free
Lite non-dairy	2 teaspoons	Free
Non dairy creamer	1 tablespoon	Free
Comet cups, waffle cones	1	Free
Condiments:		
Barbecue sauce	1 tablespoon	Free
Catsup	1 tablespoon	Free
Chili sauce	1 tablespoon	Free
Heinz 57	1 tablespoon	Free
Horseradish	3 tablespoons	Free
Mustard	1 tablespoon	Free
Pickles (except sweet)		Free
Pickle relish	1 tablespoon	Free
Soy sauce	1 tablespoon	Free
Tabasco sauce	1 tablespoon	Free
Taco sauce	1 tablespoon	Free
Teriyaki sauce	1 tablespoon	Free
Tomato sauce	2 tablespoons	Free
Worcestershire sauce	1 tablespoon	Free
Cranberries, cooked without sugar	½ cup	Free
Creamed cheese, Weight Watchers	1 tablespoon	Free
Dips:		
Picante sauce	2 tablespoons	Free
Lean cream dip, all varieties	1 tablespoon	Free

FOOD	QUANTITY	EXCHANGES
Lite dips, clam, French onion	2 tablespoons	Free
Frozen desserts:		
NutraSweet sugar-free pops	1	Free
Crystal Light Bars	1	Free
Lite Pops	1	Free
Gelatins:		
D-Zerta, low-calorie		Free
Dietetic		Free
Sugar-Free		Free
Gravies, canned:		
Au jus	¼ cup	Free
All others	2 tablespoons	Free
Jams, Jellies:		
Dietetic	Less than 20 calories per serving	Free
Low-calorie fruit spreads, sweetened with fructose	1 teaspoon	Free
Low-sugar spread	2 teaspoons	Free
Reduced-calorie	2 teaspoons	Free
Fruit spreadables, All-Fruit, Simply Fruit, Totally Fruit	1 teaspoon	Free
Mayonnaise-type salad dressing, fat-free	1 tablespoon	Free
Milk flavorings:		
Quik, sugar-free	1 heaping teaspoon	Free
Sugar-free hot cocoa mix	2 rounded scoops	Free
Molly McButter sprinkles	2 teaspoons	Free
Mrs. Dash herb and spice blends	1 teaspoon	Free
No-stick vegetable spray		Free
Onions		Free
Pimiento		Free
Postum, cereal beverage	2 teaspoons	Free
Salad dressings:		
Low-calorie	1 tablespoon	Free
Fat-free Miracle Whip	1 tablespoon	Free
No-oil mixes	2 tablespoons	Free
Non-fat dressings	3 tablespoon	Free
Reduced-calorie	1 tablespoon	Free

FOOD	QUANTITY	EXCHANGES
Salsa, all varieties	¼ cup	Free
Sauerkraut	½ cup	Free
Soups:		
Beef broth	1 cup	Free
Chicken broth	½ cup	Free
Consomme	¾ cup	Free
Sour cream:		
Light	1 tablespoon	Free
Sour Lean	1 tablespoon	Free
Sugar substitutes:		
Equal		Free
Splenda		Free
Sprinkle Sweet		Free
Sweet 'n Low		Free
Sweet One		Free
Sweet 10		Free
Syrup:		
Cary's reduced-calorie	2 tablespoons	Free
Reduced-calorie or dietetic syrups	1 tablespoon	Free
Vinegar		Free
Whipped toppings:		
Cool Whip	1 tablespoon	Free
Cool Whip Lite	2 tablespoons	Free
Dream Mix	1 tablespoon	Free
D-Zerta reduced calorie	2 tablespoons	Free
Estee	¼ cup	Free
Featherweight	¼ cup	Free
Yogurt, nonfat	2 tablespoons	Free

Spices are also free foods. The following seasonings may be used without including them as exchanges in your meal plan.

Allspice	Curry	Parsley
Angostura bitters	Dill	Pepper
Anise	Extracts, vanilla,	Poppy seed
Basil	almond, etc.	Poultry seasoning
Bay leaf	Fennel	Rosemary
Butter flavoring	Garlic, powder or salt	Saffron
Caraway	Ginger root	Sage
Cardamom	Mace	Savory
Celery salt or seed	Marjoram	Sesame seed
Chervil	Mint	Sorrel
Chili powder	Monosodium glutamate	Spice blends, premixed,
Chives	Mustard, dry	all varieties
Cinnamon	Nutmeg	Tarragon
Cloves	Onion juice, powder or salt	Tenderizers
Coriander	Oregano	Thyme
Cumin	Paprika	Turmeric

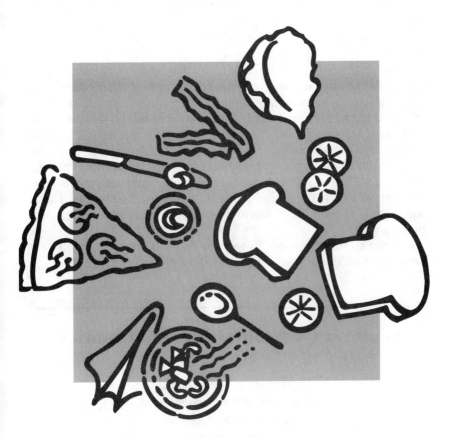

EXCHANGES FOR
COMBINATION FOODS

Many foods are a combination of foods from several of the exchange lists. By combining foods you have the advantages of the different food groups, but it sometimes makes it difficult to know how to use them in your meal plan.

Starch/bread and meat exchanges can be used to count many casseroles or mixed dishes. If you are unsure of the makeup of a combination dish, count one cup as 2 starch/bread plus 2 medium-fat meat exchanges. Depending on the ingredients, the casserole may also include a fat or a vegetable exchange. (Looks like a sandwich, doesn't it?) For example, one cup of chili, beef stew, or macaroni and beef casserole is 2 starch/bread and 2 medium fat meat exchanges. One cup of tuna noodle casserole made with cream soup is 2 starch/bread, 2 medium fat meat, and one fat exchange. This is a good rule of thumb and will allow you to add variety to your meal planning.

Some common mixed dishes are listed below. They will vary depending on the ingredients, and values given are average.

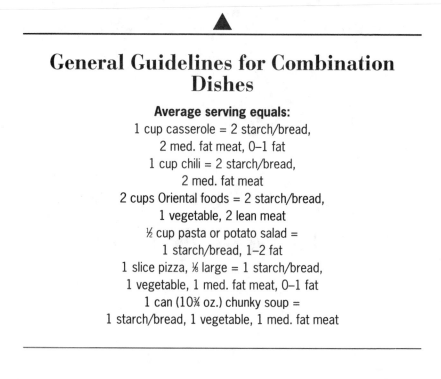

▲

General Guidelines for Combination Dishes

Average serving equals:
1 cup casserole = 2 starch/bread,
2 med. fat meat, 0–1 fat
1 cup chili = 2 starch/bread,
2 med. fat meat
2 cups Oriental foods = 2 starch/bread,
1 vegetable, 2 lean meat
½ cup pasta or potato salad =
1 starch/bread, 1–2 fat
1 slice pizza, ⅛ large = 1 starch/bread,
1 vegetable, 1 med. fat meat, 0–1 fat
1 can (10¾ oz.) chunky soup =
1 starch/bread, 1 vegetable, 1 med. fat meat

▲ EXPANDED FOOD LIST ▲

Combination Foods

FOOD	QUANTITY	EXCHANGES
Main Dishes:		
Bean soup	1 cup	1 starch/bread
		1 vegetable
		1 lean meat
Beef and vegetable stew	1 cup	1 starch/bread
		2 med. fat meat
Beef ravioli	1 cup	2 starch/bread
		1 vegetable
		1 med. fat meat
Burrito, all varieties	1 (6 oz.)	2 starch/bread
		2 med. fat meat
		1 fat
Chimichangas, all varieties	1 (6 oz.)	2 starch/bread
		1 med. fat meat
		3 fat
Creamed chipped beef	1 cup	1 starch/bread
		2 med. fat meat
		3 fat
Chicken a la king	1 cup	1 starch/bread
		2 med. fat meat
		2 fat
Chicken and dumplings	1 cup	2 starch/bread
		2 med. fat meat
		1 fat
Chicken and noodles	1 cup	2 starch/bread
		2 med. fat meat
		1 fat
Chili with beans	1 cup	2 starch/bread
		2 med. fat meat
Chow mein	1½ cup	1 starch/bread
		1 vegetable
		2 med. fat meat

FOOD	QUANTITY	EXCHANGES
Chop suey	1 cup	1 starch/bread
		3 med. fat meat
Chunky soup	1 can	1 starch/bread
	(10¾ oz.)	1 vegetable
		1 med. fat meat
Enchiladas	1	2 starch/bread
		1 med. fat meat
		1 fat
Fish cake, fried	3 pieces	1 starch/bread
		3 med. fat meat
French toast	2 slices	2 starch/bread
		2 med. fat meat
		1 fat
Hamburger Helper main dishes, ground beef	⅕ pkg, ⅕ lb	2 starch/bread
		2 med. fat meat
		1 fat
Lasagna	6 oz.	1½ starch/bread
		2 med. fat meat
Macaroni and cheese	1 cup	2 starch/bread
		1 high fat meat
Pizza, cheese or sausage	1 small slice	1 starch/bread
		1 med. fat meat
Pizza, thin crust pizza	¼ med.	2 starch/bread
		1 vegetable
		1 med. fat meat
Pizza, thick crust pizza	¼	4 starch/bread
		1 med. fat meat
Pot pies, all varieties	1 average	3 starch/bread
		1 med. fat meat
		4 fat
Quiche, all varieties	1 slice	1½ starch/bread
		2 med. fat meat
		2 fat
Rice-A-Roni	1 cup	4 starch/bread
		2 fat
Souffle, cheese or spinach	1½ cup	½ starch/bread
		2 med. fat meat
		1 fat
Spanish rice	1 cup	3 starch/bread
		1 fat

FOOD	QUANTITY	EXCHANGES
Spaghetti with meatballs and tomato sauce	1 cup	2 starch/bread 1 vegetable 2 med. fat meat
Tuna Helper main dishes	⅕ pkg, 1.3 oz. tuna	2 starch/bread 2 med. fat meat
Salads:		
Caesar salad	1 serving	2 vegetable 6 fat
Chef's salad (mixed greens, 3 Tbsp. regular dressing, 1 oz. cheese, chicken, and ham)	1 serving	1 starch/bread **or** 3 vegetable 3 med. fat meat 2 fat
Chicken salad	½ cup	2 med. fat meat 2 fat
Coleslaw	½ cup	1 vegetable 2 fat
Egg salad	½ cup	1 med. fat meat 4 fat
Pasta salads	½ cup	1½ starch/bread 1 to 2 fat
Potato salad	½ cup	1 starch/bread 1 to 2 fat
Tuna salad	½ cup	2 med. fat meat 1 fat
Waldorf salad	½ cup	1 fruit 3 fat
Sandwiches:		
Bacon, lettuce, tomato mayonnaise	1 sandwich	2 starch/bread 3 fat
Chicken, lettuce, mayonnaise .	1 sandwich	2 starch/bread 2 med. fat meat 1 fat
Chicken salad	1 sandwich	2 starch/bread 2 med. fat meat 1 fat
Club sandwich (bacon, turkey or ham, tomato, lettuce and mayonnaise on 3 slices bread)	1 sandwich	3 starch/bread 4 med. fat meat 1 fat
Corned beef	1 sandwich	2 starch/bread 3 med. fat meat

FOOD	QUANTITY	EXCHANGES
Egg salad	1 sandwich	2 starch/bread 1 med. fat meat 2 fat
Grilled cheese	1 sandwich	2 starch/bread 2 med. fat meat 2 fat
Ham salad	1 sandwich	2 starch/bread 1 med. fat meat 2 fat
Hot dog in roll	1	1½ starch/bread 1 high fat meat 2 fat
Liverwurst	1 sandwich	2 starch/bread 1 high fat meat 2 fat
Meat loaf	1 sandwich	2 starch/bread 3 med. fat meat
Peanut butter	1 sandwich	2 starch/bread 1 high fat meat 1 fat
Roast beef or pork with gravy	1 sandwich	2 starch/bread 2 med. fat meat 2 fat
Submarine sandwich or hoagie	1 large	4 starch/bread 4 med. fat meat 1 fat
Tuna salad	1 sandwich	2 starch/bread 1 med. fat meat 2 fat

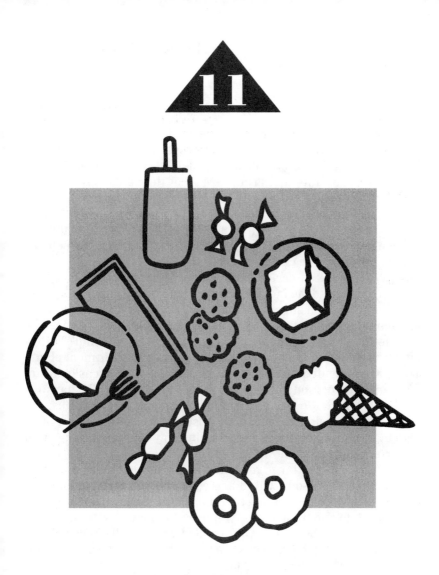

EXCHANGES FOR OCCASIONAL USE FOODS

At the tip of the pyramid, squeezed in with the fats and oils, are the sweets, with the warning "eat sparingly." When choosing foods for a healthful diet, consider the added sugars and fat in your choices from all the food groups. Most of the added sugars come from foods in the Pyramid tip—soft drinks, candy, jams, jellies, syrups, and table sugar added to foods like coffee or cereal. Added sugars are also in foods such as sweetened yogurt, chocolate milk, canned or frozen fruit with heavy syrup, ice cream, and sweetened bakery products like cakes, cookies, and pies.

These foods can occasionally be used as starch/bread or fruit exchanges despite the fact that they contain added sugars. Because they contain added sugars (and often are high in fat as well), their use should be restricted.

Dietitians are frequently asked, "What is occasional?" "How often should individuals substitute these foods in their meal plan?" These are difficult questions because what may be "occasional" for one family or person can be "frequent" for another. Perhaps the best advice is that everyone, including persons with diabetes, can benefit from avoiding foods high in sugar. These foods are often high in fat and calories as well, providing only calories without other important nutrients, known as "empty calories."

No one can eat large amounts of these foods and maintain weight, just as persons with diabetes cannot eat large amounts of these foods without elevating their blood glucose levels. However, if you choose to use these foods, you need to know how to do so correctly—how to substitute in your meal plan. You will notice the portion sizes are very small, since these foods often are concentrated sources of carbohydrates and fat.

Remember that for persons with diabetes, the goal of meal planning is to help you keep your blood glucose and fats as normal and optimal as possible. Checking your blood glucose an hour and a half after you finish a meal will help you know how these foods affect your blood glucose levels. Having your doctor check your glycosylated hemoglobin values (a test that helps evaluate your overall blood glucose levels during the past four to six weeks) and blood fats (cholesterol and triglycerides) will also help you know how well you are meeting your nutritional goals.

▲
___

General Guidelines for Sweets

One serving equals:
2" square unfrosted cake or brownie =
1 starch/bread, 1 fat
1 cookie, 3" diameter =
1 starch/bread, 0–1 fat
2 small cookies =
1 starch/bread, 0–1 fat
½ cup ice cream =
1 starch/bread, 2 fat
⅓ cup frozen yogurt =
1 starch/bread

▲ OCCASIONAL USE FOODS ▲

FOOD	QUANTITY	EXCHANGES
Brownies	2" square	1 starch/bread
		1 fat
Cakes:		
Angel food cake	½₂th cake	2 starch/bread
Applesauce spice,	½₂th cake	2 starch/bread
from mix		2 fat
Banana, from mix	½₂th cake	2 starch/bread
		2 fat
Carrot, from mix	½₂th cake	2 starch/bread
		1 fat
Commercial cake mix (chocolate,	½₂th cake	2 starch/bread
white, yellow, lemon, etc.)		2 fat

FOOD	QUANTITY	EXCHANGES
Cupcake	1	2 starch/bread 1 fat
Gingerbread, from mix	½ cake	2 starch/bread 1 fat
Pound cake, from mix	½" slice	1½ starch/bread 1 fat
Snackin', from mix	⅛ cake	2 starch/bread 1 fat
Shortcake	1 average	1 starch/bread
Cookies:		
In general, 3" diameter	1	1 starch/bread
1¾" diameter	2	1 starch/bread
Animal crackers	7	1 starch/bread
Butter cookies	4	1 starch/bread 1 fat
Chocolate chip	2, 1¾" diameter	1 starch/bread 1 fat
Chocolate wafers	3	1 starch/bread
Dinosaur cookies, mini	14	1 starch/bread ½ fat
Fig Newtons or bars	2	1½ starch/bread
Fortune cookies	2	1 starch/bread
Frookies	2	1 starch/bread 1 fat
Gingersnaps	3	1 starch/bread
Ladyfingers	2	1 starch/bread
Lorna Doone shortbread	6	1 starch/bread 1 fat
Nilla wafers	5	1 starch/bread ½ fat
Oatmeal and oatmeal raisin	2	1 starch/bread 1 fat
Oreo sandwich	2	1 starch/bread 1 fat
Peanut butter	2	1 starch/bread 1 fat
Sugar cookies	2	1 starch/bread 1 fat
Sugar wafers	2	1 starch/bread 1 fat

FOOD	QUANTITY	EXCHANGES
Vanilla wafers	6	1 starch/bread 1 fat
Chocolate syrup	2 tablespoons	1 starch/bread
Cream puff shell	1	1 starch/bread 2 fat
Custard, baked	½ cup	1 starch/bread 1 med. fat meat
Doughnuts, cake	1	1 starch/bread 1 fat
Frozen desserts:		
Frozen yogurt	⅓ cup	1 starch/bread
Fruit & cream bar	1 bar	1 starch/bread
Fruit ice	¼ cup	1 starch/bread
Fruit juice bar	1 bar	1 starch/bread
Ice cream, all flavors	½ cup	1 starch/bread 2 fat
Ice cream bars	1	1 starch/bread 2 fat
Ice milk	½ cup	1 starch/bread 1 fat
Ice milk, soft serve	½ cup	1 starch/bread 1 fat
Pudding pops	1	1 starch/bread
Sherbet	¼ cup	1 starch/bread
Sorbet	¼ cup	1 starch/bread
Sugar-free ice cream bars	1	1 starch/bread 2 fat
Sugar-free ice cream sandwiches	1	1½ starch/bread 1 fat
Gelatin desserts, all flavors	½ cup	1 starch/bread
Granola bar, plain, not chocolate coated	1	1 starch/bread 1 fat
Pie crust	⅙ crust	1 starch/bread 2 fat
Puddings:		
All varieties	½ cup	2 starch/bread 1 fat
Bread	½ cup	2½ starch/bread 1½ fat

FOOD	QUANTITY	EXCHANGES
Rice	½ cup	2 starch/bread 1 fat
Tapioca	½ cup	2 starch/bread 1 fat
Syrup:		
Maple	1 tablespoon	1 fruit
Light	2 tablespoon	1 fruit

The following foods in the amounts listed also contain 15 grams of carbohydrate and are the equivalent of one fruit exchange. They are not recommended for regular use because they contain significant amounts of refined sugars. However, persons who have diabetes and take insulin by injection may find them convenient to use to treat insulin reactions (hypoglycemia).

Butterscotch balls	3	1 fruit
Carbonated beverages	¾ cup (6 oz.)	1 fruit
Corn syrup or honey	1 tablespoon	1 fruit
Flavored ades	½ cup	1 fruit
Flavored punches	½ cup	1 fruit
Flavored fruit drinks	½ cup	1 fruit
Gelatin, regular	½ cup	1 fruit
Granulated sugar	4 teaspoons	1 fruit
Gumdrops	18 average	1 fruit
Hard candy	3 average	1 fruit
Jelly beans	9	1 fruit
Lemon drops	8	1 fruit
LifeSavers	8	1 fruit
Marshmallows	3 large	1 fruit
Maple syrup	1 tablespoon	1 fruit
Sundance beverages	5 oz.	1 fruit

PUTTING IT ALL TOGETHER: CHOOSING WHAT WE EAT

Lifestyle has a strong influence on our health—and eating is an important part of lifestyle. Fortunately, most of us can choose what we eat. Awareness of the health benefits and risks associated with various nutrients found in foods leads to an important question: "How should we eat to stay healthy?"

The Food Guide Pyramid reflects the latest scientific knowledge on nutrition and emphasizes healthy eating. The Food Guide Pyramid and the exchange lists help you put the Dietary Guidelines for Americans—advice for a healthful diet—into action. A key feature is the positive approach to meal planning. The exchange lists can make it easier to make healthy food choices.

Research has shown that control of certain dietary substances or nutrients can reduce our risk of heart disease, high blood pressure, stroke, obesity, noninsulin-dependent or type II diabetes, some forms of cancer, and cirrhosis of the liver. Furthermore, the nutritional recommendations made by the American Heart Association, American Cancer Society and National Institute of Cancer, American Diabetes Association and the Dietary Guidelines for Americans are all very similar.

If your family's eating habits need to change because someone has a high blood cholesterol level, has developed diabetes, or has a weight problem, consider yourself lucky—not deprived. You now have a special reason to pay attention to planning meals and snacks that will help your family live better today and in the future. Eating wholesome, nutritionally healthy foods will be to everyone's advantage—with or without any health problems.

What are the guidelines for good nutrition? Here's an overview of some important nutrition recommendations.

Calories

It is important for everyone to eat the amounts and types of food that meet their caloric requirements. Children and adolescents often require large numbers of calories to provide for their energy and growth requirements. They do NOT need a diet restricted in calories, but they also should not eat a diet with excessive calories in relation to their energy needs. Lean or normal weight adults also need enough calories to maintain their weight.

However, for some individuals, especially those with weight problems, a meal plan that helps them lose weight may be important. The meal plan should not be so restrictive in calories that it makes adherence impossible. Usually even moderate amounts of weight loss, 10 to 20 pounds, will improve blood glucose levels, improve blood pressure readings, and improve blood fat (cholesterol and triglyceride) levels. Cutting back 500 calories from your daily intake will normally produce a gradual weight loss. The lowest calorie intake recommended for women is 1,200 calories; 1,500 calories is the daily minimum for men. To lose more weight, increase your caloric expenditure through exercise.

Carbohydrate

The amount of carbohydrate (starches, sugars, fiber) in your diet should ideally be between 50 to 60 percent of your total calories. However, this should also be individualized for your lifestyle. A high-fiber, lower-fat diet is generally recommended. See Chapters 22 and 23 for ideas on how to do this.

Choose a diet with plenty of vegetables, fruits, and grain products which provide needed vitamins, minerals, fiber, complex carbohydrates, and sugars found naturally in foods. Use foods with added sugars only in moderation. Sugar calories are called "empty calories," meaning that they provide no important nutrients (vitamins, minerals, or fiber). A diet with lots of sugars can have too many calories and too few nutrients for most people.

Some persons with diabetes may be able to use modest amounts of added sugars in their meal plan without it affecting their blood glucose control. Different carbohydrates affect blood glucose levels differently, but it is not a matter of sugar versus starch as to how they affect blood glucose levels. First, if you choose to eat foods containing sugar, you must realize the portion sizes need to be small. Most foods containing sugar will have a considerable number of calories packed into a relatively small serving size!

Second, you need to know how to use foods containing sugar correctly. Generally foods containing sugar (cookies, cakes, ice cream, and so on) are substituted for starch/bread or fruit exchanges. See Chapter 11 for ideas on how to do this. Unfortunately, there are few foods we can eat "all we want," or in very large portions, without affecting weight or blood glucose control!

Protein

Generally, most Americans consume between 12 to 20 percent of their calories from protein; it would be unusual if this were not sufficient. The majority of Americans consume two to three times as much protein as they actually need. This is also true for persons with diabetes.

Fat

Choose a diet low in fat, saturated fat, and cholesterol to reduce your risk of heart disease and certain types of cancer. Because fat contains over twice the calories of an equal amount of carbohydrate or protein, a diet low in fat can also help you maintain a reasonable weight.

The leading causes of death for all Americans are related to diseases of the heart and blood vessels. The three main risk factors for this are high blood cholesterol levels, high blood pressure, and smoking. Diets high in fat, especially saturated fat, and cholesterol contribute to elevated blood cholesterol. By cutting back on saturated fats and cholesterol you can lower your blood cholesterol levels. It is recommended that 30 percent of your calories come from fat, and dietary cholesterol be limited to 300 mg per day. Try to reduce your intake of saturated fats and/or replace it with limited amounts of unsaturated fats. See Chapter 23 for ideas on how to do this.

There is also evidence that unsaturated fats from fish, called fish oils or "omega 3s," may be beneficial in lowering triglycerides and possibly cholesterol. Fish found in cold waters, "fatty" fish, and even shellfish are good sources of these fish oils and should be eaten a couple of times a week. Fish oil capsules are not recommended.

Salt (Sodium)

Too much sodium (a major component of salt) is a prime suspect in the development of high blood pressure (hypertension), especially in persons who have a family history of high blood pressure. Because of this, it is recommended that sodium intake be kept to less than 3,000 milligrams (mg) of sodium per day. For persons who have hypertension, sodium intake should be limited to about 2,400 mg per day. One teaspoon of salt provides about 2,300 mg of sodium.

Be careful about the use of salt while cooking and at the table and foods that are high in sodium. This includes cured meats, luncheon meats, and many cheeses, most canned soups and vegetables, and soy sauce. Look for lower salt and no-salt-added versions of these products at the supermarket.

Food labels list the amount of sodium in foods in milligrams per serving. Look for foods that have fewer than 400 mg of sodium per single serving, or meals or entrees that have fewer than 800 mg of sodium per serving. See Chapter 24 for additional information on sodium.

Nonnutritive Sweeteners

Nonnutritive sweeteners, also called high intensity or low-caloric sweeteners, made from aspartame (Equal® or NutraSweet®), saccharin (Sweet 'n Low or Sugar Twin), or acesulfame-K (Sweet One™ or Sunette™), are safe to use. Some of these products may contribute a very minimal amount of calories, but the amount is negligible. See Chapter 25 for more information on sweeteners.

Alcohol

Everyone should be aware of the dangers of too much alcohol. Drinking alcohol can be the cause of many health problems and accidents and can lead to addiction. But people who have diabetes and take insulin or an oral medication should also be aware that alcohol consumed without food can cause too low a blood sugar level (hypoglycemia). Nonetheless, if you choose to drink an occasional alcoholic beverage, you can usually do so safely. See Chapter 31 for guidelines.

If You Have Diabetes—

The goal of meal planning is to help you keep your blood glucose levels in as good control, or near normal, as possible and to keep blood fats (cholesterol and triglycerides) in an ideal range.

For people who use insulin, the best way to do this is to eat as consistently as possible—approximately the same amount of foods at the same times each day. By eating consistently and by monitoring your blood glucose levels, insulin therapy can be integrated into your food habits. But if it is not known when and how much food you usually eat, it is difficult to know the kind and amount of insulin you require.

For people with Type II diabetes being controlled by diet alone, diet and oral medications, or diet and insulin, the best way to help you meet your goals is by weight management. Even small amounts of weight loss—10 to 20 pounds—can improve blood glucose levels and reduce the need for oral medications or insulin. But even without weight loss, making better food choices, learning new eating behaviors, and exercise can be helpful.

And Finally—

As you think about healthy eating and how your family will follow the same nutritional guidelines, keep these goals in mind:

Good food, good health, and good taste.

Too often we equate a diet rich in fat, cholesterol, sugar, calories, and salt with good tasting food. However, this is not necessarily true. Healthy food can and does taste good!

Poor eating habits are risk factors for many of the chronic diseases affecting Americans today. The happy truth is that with gradual and moderate changes in our eating habits, we can live much better and probably longer—and we'll look better, too.

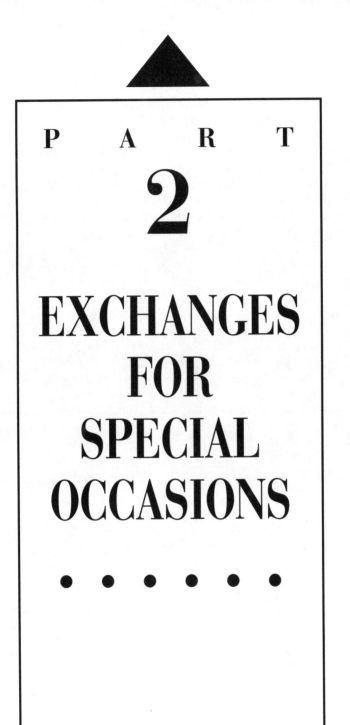

2

EXCHANGES FOR SPECIAL OCCASIONS

● ● ● ● ●

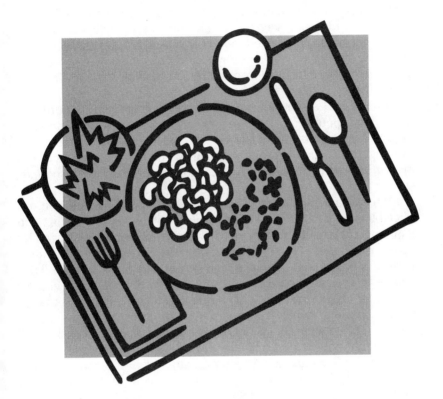

EXCHANGES
VEGETARIAN

Many people are varying their diets these days with vegetarian dishes and meals. Vegetarianism is not new; vegetarianism or near-vegetarianism has been practiced for thousands of years. People may choose a vegetarian diet for health, religious, ethnic, philosophical, ecological, or economic reasons. Others simply enjoy the taste of a variety of new or unfamiliar foods. Whatever your motivation, if you have chosen or are considering a vegetarian way of eating, you will find this chapter helpful.

Traditional American meal planning is based on main dishes using meat, poultry, or fish. Vegetarians use alternative sources of protein from plants. Some are very similar to meats, others less so. In a vegetarian diet legumes and grains and often soy products and meat analogs (meat substitutes, usually made from soy products) supply most of the protein.

Vegetarians tend to use more whole grain products and legumes (dried beans, peas, lentils) than nonvegetarians. Whole grains and legumes are excellent sources of vitamins, minerals, and protein. They are also excellent sources of fiber. Meals with vegetable proteins in place of meat can be low in fat unless a lot of high-fat dairy products, such as cheese, whole milk, butter, or cream, are eaten.

There are several types of vegetarians. *Vegans*, or strict vegetarians, eat only foods from plant sources, such as fruits, grains, legumes (dried beans, peas, lentils), nuts, and seeds, and exclude all foods of animal origin. *Lactovegetarians* eat plant foods plus dairy products but exclude meat, poultry, fish, and eggs. *Lacto-ovovegetarians* eat plant foods plus both dairy products and eggs but exclude meat, poultry, and fish.

All vegetarians, even vegans, can have healthy diets, if they select their foods carefully to provide a balance of essential amino acids (the building blocks of protein), adequate sources of vitamins and minerals, and sufficient calories.

Both the quality and quantity of the protein we eat is important. Animal proteins, such as meat and milk, are called *complete proteins* because they supply all the amino acids needed in the body. Of the 20 or so amino acids that make up protein, nine cannot be manufactured by the body. They are called *essential amino acids* because they must be supplied in the diet. Many foods, however, are lacking in one or more of the essential amino acids. For example, most plant foods, such as legumes and wheat, are not complete because they are low in one or two of the essential amino acids. To be complete proteins, they must be combined with other proteins that supplement or supply the missing amino acids. In a vegetarian diet, plant proteins are combined to complement each other in meeting the body's protein needs without using animal foods.

It sounds complicated, but it's actually quite simple. By combining different common protein-rich plant foods at the same meal, or within a short time of the meal, plant proteins can meet the body's needs for essential amino acids. For example, lentils combined with wheat or rice, or any legume combined with grains or cereals, are now complete proteins. This is what happens when you eat baked beans with brown bread. Other examples of complementary protein combinations are:

   corn/beans (cornbread or corn tortillas with chili beans)
   beans/rice (red beans and rice)
   peas/rye (split pea soup with rye bread)
   nuts/wheat (peanut butter on bread)

By mixing grains with legumes or low-fat dairy products, you complete proteins. Plant proteins may be combined with milk, cheese, or egg to provide complete proteins. Grain products can include brown or white rice, barley, pasta, kasha, whole-grain breads, and cereals. Legumes include lentils, all beans, chickpeas, tofu and other soy products. Low-fat dairy products include skim or 1% milk, low-fat or nonfat yogurt and cheese with 5 grams or less fat per ounce. Some examples are:

   cereals/milk (breakfast cereal with milk)
   pasta/cheese (macaroni and cheese)
   bread/cheese (cheese sandwich)
   beans/cheese (tamale pie)

Soybeans and soy products are, however, complete proteins by themselves. Products made from soy are available and are comparable in protein quality to meat. They can be substituted or used for meat without changing the rest of the menu. Included in this meat analog list are steaks, chops, wieners, and hamburger-style products. They add interest and variety to meals but are not essential for a well-balanced diet.

Legumes and some commercial vegetarian meat substitutes made with soy and/or wheat are higher in carbohydrate but lower in fat than meat. In these cases, a starch/bread exchange may also need to be omitted. For example, one cup of cooked legumes is the equivalent of 2 starch/bread and 1 lean meat exchange or ½ cup cooked legumes is the equivalent of 1 starch/bread and ½ lean meat exchange.

A one-cup serving of cooked legumes with a complementary plant protein or small amount of animal protein (milk, cheese, eggs) nutritionally replaces a three-ounce portion of meat, fish, or poultry.

If you plan to substitute vegetarian menus occasionally in your meal plan, substitutes for meat exchanges may be chosen from nuts or nut butters, eggs, cheeses, legumes, soy beans, or soy substitutes such as tofu. If nuts or nut butters are used, fat exchanges must be omitted, since nuts contain more fat than meat. Eggs, cottage cheese or skim milk cheeses, tofu, or soy beans can be substituted for meat without other changes, since they have about the same exchange value.

The following are some meal suggestions that are quick and easy to prepare.

Breakfast:

Many traditional breakfast foods are good choices. For instance: whole-grain, ready-to-eat or hot cereal and skim or 1% milk; waffles or pancakes with fruit and a dollop of low-fat or nonfat yogurt; whole-grain breads, rolls, bagels, or English muffins with low-fat cheese, such as 1% cottage cheese, farmers cheese, or part-skim mozzarella. Low-fat, cholesterol-free egg substitutes are also available.

Lunch:

Many good meatless soups are an option: lentil, bean, split pea, vegetable, or barley, as well as cold soups like borscht or gazpacho. They can be eaten with low-fat or nonfat plain yogurt or artificially sweetened fruited yogurt and low-fat, whole-grain breads and crackers. Plain or vegetable pizza is another good choice, but adding the extra cheese topping adds extra fat calories.

Dinner:

Pasta (especially the whole-grain variety) with a tomato-based sauce, added vegetables such as beans, mushrooms, onions, peppers, and some grated cheese, or lasagna made with a meatless tomato sauce, spinach, and ricotta and part-skim or low-fat mozzarella cheese are hearty and low-fat dishes. Whole grains such as barley, kasha, and brown rice can be mixed with beans and chickpeas, corn kernels, and diced peppers, and served with low-fat or nonfat yogurt. Mexican soft bean-filled enchiladas and burritos accompanied by rice and beans are other good choices. To cut back on fat, use sour cream, shredded cheese, guacamole, lard, and fried tortillas sparingly. Supplement choices with fruit or fruit juice, or add fruit or juice to any of the low-fat or nonfat yogurts.

▲ EXPANDED EXCHANGES ▲

Vegetarian Diet

FOOD	QUANTITY	EXCHANGES
Starch/Bread:		
Arabic bread, Syrian bread	½ of a 2 oz. loaf	1 starch/bread
Barley, cooked	⅓ cup	1 starch/bread
Brewer's yeast	3 tablespoons	1 starch/bread 1 lean meat
Brown rice, cooked	⅓ cup	1 starch/bread
Buckwheat flour, dark or light	3 tablespoons	1 starch/bread
Buckwheat groats, kasha, cooked	½ cup	1 starch/bread
Bulgur, cooked	½ cup	1 starch/bread
Bulgur, dry	2 tablespoons	1 starch/bread
Carob flour	2 tablespoons	1 starch/bread
Couscous, cooked	⅓ cup	1 starch/bread

FOOD	QUANTITY	EXCHANGES
Falafel 2" diameter	3 patties,	1 starch/bread 1 med. fat meat 2 fat
Hummus	⅓ cup	1 starch/bread 1½ fat
Millet, cooked	⅔ cup	1 starch/bread
Miso	3 tablespoons	1 starch/bread ½ med. fat meat
Oats, cooked	½ cup	1 starch/bread
Pocket bread, pita 4½" diameter	1	1 starch/bread
Pocket bread, pita 6½" diameter	½ loaf (1 oz.)	1 starch/bread
Rice cakes, all varieties	2	1 starch/bread
Rye flour	3 tablespoons	1 starch/bread
Split pea soup	1 cup	2 starch/bread 1 lean meat
Soybean flour, full-fat	½ cup	1 starch/bread 2 med. fat meat
Soybean flour, low-fat	½ cup	1 starch/bread 3 lean meat
Tempeh	½ cup	1 starch/bread 2 lean meat
Wheat berries, cooked	⅔ cup	1 starch/bread
Wheat bran, toasted, Kretschmer	1 oz.	1 starch/bread
Wheat germ, toasted	¼ cup	1 starch/bread 1 lean meat
Wild rice, cooked	½ cup	1 starch/bread
Lean Meat:		
Cheeses, see Chapter Four		
Bacon substitute	2 tablespoons	1 lean meat
Soy grits, raw	2 tablespoons	1 lean meat
Textured vegetable protein	¾ oz.	1 lean meat ½ starch/bread
Dried Beans and Peas, cooked		
Black beans, turtle beans	1 cup	2 starch/bread 1 lean meat

FOOD	QUANTITY	EXCHANGES
Black-eyed peas, cowpeas	1 cup	2 starch/bread 1 lean meat
Broad beans, faba beans	⅔ cup	2 starch/bread 1 lean meat
Calico	1 cup	2 starch/bread 1 lean meat
Garbanzo, chickpeas	⅔ cup	2 starch/bread 1 lean meat
Kidney	1 cup	2 starch/bread 1 lean meat
Lentils	1 cup	2 starch/bread 1 lean meat
Lima	1 cup	2 starch/bread 1 lean meat
Mung	2 cups	1 starch/bread 1 lean meat
Navy	⅔ cup	2 starch/bread 1 lean meat
Pinto	⅔ cup	2 starch/bread 1 lean meat
Split peas	⅔ cup	2 starch/bread 1 lean meat

Medium Fat Meat:
Cheeses, see Chapter Four

Natto	½ cup	2 med. fat meat 1 starch/bread
Soybeans, cooked	⅓ cup	1 med. fat meat ½ starch/bread
Tofu	½ cup	1 med. fat meat

High Fat Meat:
Cheeses, see Chapter Four
Nuts:

Almonds	¼ cup (1 oz.)	1 high fat meat 1 fat
Brazil nuts	¼ cup (1 oz.)	1 high fat meat 2 fat
Butternuts	¼ cup (1 oz.)	1 high fat meat 1 fat
Peanuts, roasted	¼ cup (1 oz.)	1 high fat meat 1 fat

FOOD	QUANTITY	EXCHANGES
Pecans	¼ cup (1 oz.)	1 high fat meat 1 fat
Pignolias, pine nuts	2 tablespoons	1 high fat meat 1 fat
Pistachio	47 nuts (1 oz.)	1 high fat meat 1 fat
Walnuts	16–20 halves (1 oz.)	1 high fat meat 1 fat
Peanut butter	1 tablespoon	1 high fat meat
Seeds:		
Pumpkin or squash	¼ cup	1 high fat meat 1 fat
Sesame	¼ cup	1 high fat meat 1 fat
Sunflower	¼ cup	1 high fat meat 1 fat
Sunflowers with hulls	½ cup	1 high fat meat 1 fat
Vegetable Protein Foods*		
Worthington Foods:		
Bolono, frozen	2 slices	1 lean meat
Vegetarian burger, canned	½ cup	½ starch/bread 2 lean meat
Chicken, frozen	2 slices	1 med. fat meat 1 fat
Chili, canned	⅔ cup	1 starch/bread 1 med. fat meat 1 fat
Choplets, canned	2 slices	2 lean meat
Corned beef, frozen	4 slices	½ starch/bread 1 med. fat meat
Country stew	9½ oz. can	1 starch/bread 1 vegetable 1 med. fat meat 1 fat
Cutlets, canned	1½ slices	2 lean meat
Dinner roast, frozen	2 slices(3 oz.)	1 high fat meat

*Brand names of meat analogs are Worthington, LaLoma, Morningstar Farms, and Natural Touch. Additional information is available from: Worthington Foods, Inc., 900 Proprietors Road, Worthington, Ohio 43085.

FOOD	QUANTITY	EXCHANGES
Non-meat balls, canned	3 pieces	1 high fat meat
Prime stakes	1 piece	½ starch/bread
		1 med. fat meat
		1 fat
Prosage links, frozen	2 links	1 high fat meat
Salami, meatless, frozen	2 slices	½ starch/bread
		1 lean meat
Smoked beef, frozen	3 slices	½ starch/bread
		1 med. fat meat
Smoked turkey, frozen	4 slices	2 lean meat
Tuno, frozen	2 oz.	1 high fat meat
Turkee slices, canned	2 slices	1 med. fat meat
		1 fat
Vegetable skallops, canned	½ cup	2 lean meat
Vegetarian beef or Chicken pie, frozen	1 pie	3 starch/bread
		4 fat
Vegetarian egg roll	1 roll	1 starch/bread
		1 vegetable
		1 fat
Wham, frozen	3 slices	2 med. fat meat
La Loma:		
Big franks, canned	1 frank	2 lean meat
Chicken, fried, frozen	1 piece (2 oz.)	2 med. fat meat
		1 fat
Corn dogs,frozen	1 dog	1 starch/bread
		2 med. fat meat
Griddle steak, frozen	1 steak (2 oz.)	2 lean meat
Nuteena, canned	½" slice	1 med. fat meat
		2 fat
Savory meatballs, frozen	7 meatballs	3 lean meat
		1 vegetable
Swiss steak, canned	1 piece	2 med. fat meat
		1 vegetable
Vege-burger, canned	½ cup	3 lean meat
Morningstar Farms:		
Breakfast links, frozen	2 links	1 med. fat meat
Breakfast pattie, frozen	1 pattie	1 high fat meat
Breakfast strips	3 strips	2 fat
Scramblers, frozen	¼ cup	1 lean meat

FOOD	QUANTITY	EXCHANGES
Natural Touch:		
Dinner entree, frozen	1 patty	3 med. fat meat
Lentil rice loaf, frozen	2½" slice	1 med. fat meat
		1 fat
Vegetarian chili,	⅔ cup	1 starch/bread
canned		2 med. fat meat
Vegetable:		
Bamboo shoots, cooked	½ cup	1 vegetable
Bean sprouts,	1 cup raw **or**	1 vegetable
alfalfa, mung,	¾ cup cooked	
soy		
Carrot juice	¼ cup	1 vegetable
Seaweed, cooked	½ cup	1 vegetable
Water chestnuts, canned	6 whole	1 vegetable
Milk:		
Goat milk	1 cup	1 skim milk
		1½ fat
Kefir	1 cup	1 skim milk
		2 fat
Soy milk, fortified	1 cup	½ skim milk
		1 fat
Yogurt, lite	6–8 oz.	1 skim milk
Yogurt, fruit flavored,	6–8 oz.	1 skim milk
sweetened with NutraSweet		
Fat:		
Bacon, simulated	2 strips	1 fat
meat product		
Lecithin	2 teaspoons	1 fat
Tahini sesame paste	½ tablespoon	1 fat
Free:		
Carob powder	1 tablespoon	free
Sprouts	½ cup	free

Word List

Brewer's yeast: A savory flavoring in powdered form used as a supplement in cooking. It does not rise like regular yeast.

Buckwheat: A bushlike plant. Buckwheat seeds are called groats, coarse ground groats are grits, and finely ground groats are buckwheat flour.

Hummus: A spread made from pureed garbanzo beans (chickpeas), tahini, lemon juice, olive oil, and garlic.

Kasha: Cooked or roasted groats.

Kefir: A cultured dairy product that is similar to milk.

Legumes: Dried beans such as kidney, garbanzo, navy, pinto, lima, soybeans, peanuts, black-eyed peas, chickpeas, and lentils.

Meat analogs: Vegetable protein foods that duplicate the flavor, texture, and appearance of meat.

Miso: Soybean paste.

Soymeat: Spun soy protein products. The cheese-like curd from soybeans is sent through many mechanical manipulations in order to obtain the texture of the final product.

Tahini: Sesame seed paste.

Tempeh: Soybean derivative; contains protein and carbohydrates.

Tofu: Soft unripened cheese-like curd made from soybeans.

SAMPLE MENU

▲ Lacto-Ovovegetarian ▲

	Menu	Exchanges
Breakfast:	2 slices whole wheat toast	3 starch/bread
	½ cup cooked oats	
	½ cup orange juice	1 fruit
	1 cup skim milk	1 milk
	2 tsp. margarine	2 fat
Snack:	1 apple or 6 whole	1 fruit or
	wheat crackers	starch/bread
Lunch:	1 pita bread, ½ cup	2 starch/bread
	garbanzo spread	
	(1 lean meat from garbanzo	2 meat
	spread)	
	¼ cup cottage cheese	
	diced tomatoes, shredded	0–1 vegetable
	lettuce, diced onions	
	1 medium orange	1 fruit
	8 oz. artificially sweetened	1 milk
	fruited yogurt	
	1 tsp. tahini paste	1 fat
Snack:	4 squares RyKrisp	1 starch/bread
	½ banana	1 fruit
Dinner:	½ cup spaghetti	3 starch/bread
	(1 starch/bread)	
	1 cup lentil spaghetti sauce	2 meat
	(2 starch/bread, 2 lean meat,	1 vegetable
	1 vegetable)	
	green salad with sprouts	1 vegetable
	1 slice pineapple with juice	1 fruit
	2 Tbsp. low-calorie dressing	1 fat
Snack:	3 cups popcorn	1 starch/bread
	1 oz. low-fat cheese	1 meat
Total:	1,900 calories	260 gms carbohydrate (55%)
		90 gms protein (19%)
		55 gms fat (26%)

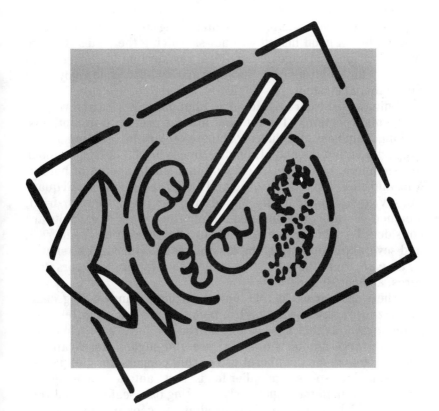

EXCHANGES WITH
CHOPSTICKS

Many Americans enjoy the richness and diversity of healthful ethnic foods. Heading this list are Asian foods—Chinese, Japanese, Thai, and Vietnamese. Interesting spices and ingredients help maintain good health without sacrificing the tastes that are part of various heritages. Many local restaurants featuring Asian foods or ethnic entrees from the supermarket allow us to enjoy these international cuisines.

Chinese dishes are based on an abundance of rice and vegetables, small portions of meat, and low-fat preparation methods, making them healthful choices. Chinese cooking involves much food preparation, but the actual cooking time is brief. Cooking methods are steaming, boiling, or stir-frying in a small amount of hot fat. Milk and cheese are rarely used and meats are used in small quantities. Vegetables seldom are served raw; they are usually stir-fried, steamed, or added to soups just minutes before serving. Fruits are considered a delicacy. A main meal usually consists of a soup, rice, and several platters of vegetables and meats which can be shared by all who are at the table. Meals include a variety of flavors, textures, and cooking methods.

There are four schools of Chinese cooking: Peking cooking, characterized by the use of garlic, leeks, scallions, noodles, and dumplings; Shanghai, specializing in "red-cooking," a form of braising with large amounts of soy sauce and sugar; Szechwan and Hunan, famous for the liberal use of chili peppers and hot pepper sauces, and for spicier and oilier foods; and Cantonese cooking, the least greasy of all the regional styles, using fish, seafoods, and vegetables. Chicken broth often is used as the cooking medium and sugar may be added as a flavoring ingredient. A Cantonese specialty is dim sum, which are dumplings stuffed with pork, shrimp, beef, sweet paste, or preserves and steamed or deep-fried and often served at a brunch.

Look for foods cooked using the stir-fry method, such as chicken with broccoli, shrimp with Chinese vegetables; or by steaming, such as dim sum selections, steamed dumplings.

Most Japanese cuisine with its emphasis on fresh vegetables and fruits and meals prepared with little fat fits into a healthy lifestyle . The basis for much of its flavor, however, is soy sauce (shoyu). This salty condiment may be a problem if you are limiting your sodium intake.

Japanese main dishes use a large variety of vegetables, along with many kinds of fish or small amounts of meat, and are seasoned with soy sauce and/or miso sauce, a soybean product. White rice is the staple food item and a variety of fresh fruit is eaten.

Deep-fat frying of fish, shellfish, and vegetables (tempura) is one of the few times when fat is used in food preparation. Look for steamed or grilled (Kushiyaki) vegetable, fish, shellfish, or skinless poultry dishes with a little tempura dipping sauce on the side. Also popular are simple cakes and cookies, made of sugar and rice flour, that contain little or no fat. Usually desserts are not part of a meal.

Thai meals also use rice as the staple and dishes that incorporate vegetables, often four to six different kinds. Smaller portions of beef, pork, poultry, and seafood (shrimp, scallops, squid, and clams) are common. Look for stir-fried, steamed, sauteed, boiled, marinated, grilled, and barbecued items on the menu. Be careful of foods fried in lard or prepared with coconut milk or cream.

The spicing and flavoring of Thai food is not as dependent on soy sauce as other Asian cuisines. Instead, chili sauce or crushed dried chilies, Thai spices, curry, and hot sauces add spice and "fire" to foods.

Vietnamese foods share many similarities with other Southeastern Asian countries. As with Chinese and Japanese cuisines the staple foods are rice, soybean products, and tea. In general, Vietnamese dishes are often lighter because vegetables are the primary ingredient. Rice products, such as noodles (sticks), paper, and flour, are used extensively. In Vietnamese cookery, rice paper is used as egg roll (spring rolls) or wonton wrappers. The moistened rice paper may be wrapped around a variety of meats, fish, vegetables, and herbs and then deep-fried. Foods are commonly stir-fried, simmered, or boiled. Soup may accompany every meal.

In Asian countries the traditional eating utensils are chopsticks and a porcelain spoon used for soup. It is considered bad manners to eat rice with the bowl resting on the table; instead, it should be raised to the mouth. With a little practice you can also become proficient at using chopsticks. Chopsticks, a boon because they extend the "reach," are made of bamboo, wood, plastic, ivory, or even silver. Although chopsticks may be difficult to use at first, they can be mastered quickly with practice. A good way to learn is to pick up and hold peanuts, one at a time! All and all, new tastes and chopsticks can add up to a remarkable dining experience.

▲ EXPANDED EXCHANGES ▲

Asian Cooking

FOOD	QUANTITY	EXCHANGES
Starch/Bread:		
Arrowroot starch	2 tablespoons	1 starch/bread
Bow (Chinese steamed dough)	1 small or ⅔ medium	1 starch/bread
Cellophane noodles, cooked	¾ cup	1 starch/bread
Chow mein noodles	½ cup	1 starch/bread 1 fat
Chestnuts	4 large, 6 small	1 starch/bread
Cornstarch	2 tablespoons	1 starch/bread
Congee rice soup	¾ cup	1 starch/bread
Egg roll wrapper	2	1 starch/bread
Fried rice	⅓ cup	1 starch/bread 2 fat
Ginkgo seeds	½ cup	1 starch/bread
Glutinous rice	⅓ cup	1 starch/bread
Lotus root	10 slices	1 starch/bread
Miso	3 tablespoons	1 starch/bread
	½ cup	2½ starch/bread 1 med. fat meat
Mung beans	⅔ cup	1 starch/bread
Mung bean noodles	¾ cup	1 starch/bread
Poi (taro, cooked)	⅓ cup	1 starch/bread
Rice, cooked (loosely packed)	⅓ cup	1 starch/bread

FOOD	QUANTITY	EXCHANGES
Rice noodles, vermicelli, cooked	½ cup	1 starch/bread
Rice soup	¾ cup	1 starch/bread
Wonton wrappers (3" x 3")	4	1 starch/bread
Wonton, fried	3	1 starch/bread 4 fat
Wonton soup, canned	1 cup	½ starch/bread
Wheat fritters	1	1 starch/bread
Yard-long beans, pods, and seeds	½ cup	1 starch/bread
Lean Meat:		
Abalone	1 oz.	1 lean meat
Chicken wings	1 wing	1 lean meat
Red mung beans	⅔ cup	1 lean meat 2 starch/bread
Horse beans, broad beans	⅔ cup	1 lean meat 2 starch/bread
Octopus	2 oz.	1 lean meat
Shrimp, dried	10 (½ oz)	1 lean meat
Squid	½ cup (2 oz.)	1 lean meat
Medium Fat Meat:		
Duck feet	3	1 med. fat meat
Egg flower soup	2 cups	1 med. fat meat
Fish maw	2 oz.	1 med. fat meat
Oxtail	1 oz.	1 med. fat meat
Tofu	½ cup (4 oz.)	1 med. fat meat
High Fat Meat:		
Anchovies	10	1 high fat meat
Chinese sausage	½ (1 oz.)	1 high fat meat
Eel	1 oz.	1 high fat meat
Pork feet	2 oz.	1 high fat meat
Preserved duck egg	1 egg	1 high fat meat
Vegetable:		
Amaranth or Chinese spinach, cooked	½ cup	1 vegetable
Arrowroot, 2" diameter	1	1 vegetable
Bok choy, cooked	1 cup	1 vegetable
Bamboo shoots, canned	½ cup	1 vegetable

FOOD	QUANTITY	EXCHANGES
Bean sprouts	1 cup raw **or** ¾ cup cooked	1 vegetable
Chayote (pear squash)	½ medium	1 vegetable
Chinese cabbage	2 cups raw **or** 1 cup cooked	1 vegetable
Corn, baby, canned	½ cup	1 vegetable
Daikon (Chinese radish)	1 cup	1 vegetable
Ginger root	¼ cup	1 vegetable
Kohlrabi	⅔ cup	1 vegetable
Leeks (Chinese onion)	½ cup **or** 2 medium	1 vegetable
Bitter melon	½ cup	1 vegetable
Fuzzy melon	½ cup	1 vegetable
Miso	1 tablespoon	1 vegetable
Button or straw mushrooms	½ cup	1 vegetable
Dried black mushrooms	¼ cup	1 vegetable
Mustard leaves	½ cup	1 vegetable
Seaweed laver, soaked	½ cup	1 vegetable
Seahair, soaked	½ cup	1 vegetable
Snow peas, sugar peas, sweet peas, peapods	½ cup	1 vegetable
Taro root	¼ cup	1 vegetable
Fruit:		
Apple pear, Asian pear	1	1 fruit
Dried salted apricots	6 halves	1 fruit
Almond cookie	2	1 fruit **or** 1 starch/bread
Fortune cookie	1 large **or** 2 small	1 fruit **or** 1 starch/bread
Carambola (star fruit)	1½	1 fruit
Red dates	6	1 fruit
Guava, fresh	½ cup **or** 1½	1 fruit
Kumquats, fresh	5	1 fruit
Longans, raw	30	1 fruit
canned	¾ cup	1 fruit
Loquats	12	1 fruit
Lychees, canned,	½ cup	1 fruit
fresh or dried	10	1 fruit
Mango, small, fresh	½	1 fruit

FOOD	QUANTITY	EXCHANGES
Papaya, fresh	¾ cup	1 fruit
Persimmon, raw	2 medium	1 fruit
Persimmon, Japanese	½ medium	1 fruit
Pomelo, raw	¾ cup	1 fruit
Fat:		
Chicken fat or pork fat	1 teaspoon	1 fat
Coconut milk	1 tablespoon	1 fat
Coconut, grated	2 tablespoons	1 fat
Macadamia nuts	3	1 fat
Pork, cured	1" cube	1 fat
Sesame or peanut oil	1 teaspoon	1 fat
Sesame paste	1½ teaspoon	1 fat
Sesame seeds	1 tablespoon	1 fat
Watermelon seeds	⅓ oz.	1 fat
Free:		
Coriander (Chinese parsley)		
Curry		
Fish sauce		
Garlic		
Ginger		
Green onion		
Hot mustard		
Soy sauce		
Star anise		
Vinegar		
Combination Dishes:		
Beef and Vegetables	2 cups	2 starch/bread 2 med. fat meat 1 vegetable
Chicken or Shrimp and Vegetables	2 cups	2 starch/bread 2 lean meat 1 vegetable
Chop Suey	1½ cup	1 starch/bread 3 med. fat meat
Chow Luny Aas (lobster tails in garlic sauce)	¾ cup	3 med. fat meat 1 fat
Chow Mein, beef, pork, or chicken	2 cups	2 starch/bread 2–3 med. fat meat 1 vegetable

FOOD	QUANTITY	EXCHANGES
Dim Sum		
Har-Gow	3 pieces	½ starch/bread
		½ med. fat meat
Siu-Mai	2 pieces	½ starch/bread
		1 med. fat meat
Gow-Gee	3 pieces	1 starch/bread
		1 med. fat meat
War-Tip	2 pieces	½ starch/bread
		1 med. fat meat
Egg Drop Soup	1 cup	Free
Egg Foo Yong	1 medium patty	2 med. fat meat
		1 vegetable
		2 fat
Egg Foo Yong Sauce	¼ cup	1 vegetable
Egg Roll, chicken, pork, or shrimp	1 small roll	1 starch/bread
		1 fat
Fried Rice (rice, meat, eggs, onion)	1 cup	2 starch/bread
		1 med. fat meat
		2 fat
Fung Gawn Aar (shrimp, chicken liver, mushrooms in chicken broth)	1 cup	3 med. fat meat
		2 fat
Mock Duck	¾ cup	1 starch/bread
		2 lean meat
Moo Goo Gai Pan	2 cups	1 starch/bread
		2–3 med. fat meat
		1 vegetable
		0–1 fat
Mum Yee Mein (braised noodles, chicken breast, mushrooms, chestnuts, Chinese peas)	1 cup	2 starch/bread
		2 med. fat meat
		1 fat
Pepper Steak	1 cup	1 starch/bread
		3 med. fat meat
		1 vegetable
Rumaki (chicken livers, water chestnuts, wrapped in bacon)	2 pieces	1 med. fat meat
		1 fat
Shiu Mi (chopped chestnuts, chives, and pork wrapped in thin noodles)	2 pieces	½ starch/bread
		½ fat

FOOD	QUANTITY	EXCHANGES
Sukiyaki	1½ cup	3 med. fat meat
		1 fat
Sweet and Sour Pork	1½ cup	2 starch/bread
		2 med. fat meat
		2 fruit
with rice	⅓ cup	1 starch/bread
Wonton, boiled	4	1 starch/bread
		1 med. fat meat
		1 fat
Wonton Soup	2 won tons and broth	1 starch/bread
		1 fat

Word List

Amaranth: Also known as Chinese spinach, it is usually stir-fried.

Bean curd, tofu: Smooth, creamy, custard-like product, made by pureeing soybeans.

Bean sprouts: Tiny white shoots with pale green hoods.

Bitter melon: Cucumber-like vegetable with a bumpy green surface and bitter flavor.

Black mushrooms: Dried fungi also known as Chinese or winter mushrooms, they are used extensively in Chinese cooking.

Bok choy: Also known as Chinese chard, it has broad white or greenish-white stalks and loose, dark-green leaves.

Carambola: Glossy, yellow pods marked with five longitudinal ribs that form a star shape when the fruit is sliced.

Cellophane noodles: Hard, opaque, fine white noodles made from ground mung beans.

Chili paste: Condiment made with mashed chili peppers, vinegar, and garlic.

Coconut milk: A liquid extracted from grating fresh coconut meat; not the liquid inside the coconut.

Congee: A thin rice gruel.

Coriander:	Also known as cilantro or Chinese parsley, it has a pungent, musky flavor.
Dim sum:	Steamed or fried dumplings stuffed with meat, seafood, and/or vegetables, sweet paste or preserves.
Duck feet:	Duck feet braised in soy sauce, sugar, wine, salt, monosodium glutamate and spices.
Duck eggs:	Duck eggs soaked in brine for 30 to 40 days.
Duck sauce:	Also known as plum sauce, made by blending plums, apricots, vinegar, and sugar.
Egg roll:	Minced or shredded meat and/or seafood and vegetables wrapped in egg roll wrapper and deep-fried.
Fish maw:	Dried and deep-fried stomach lining of fish.
Fish sauce:	A sauce made by fermenting small, salted fish in wooden casks for several months and draining the liquid.
Ginkgo nuts or seeds:	Small fruit of Ginkgo tree with tough, beige-colored shells and ivory-colored nuts.
Hoisin sauce:	Also known as Chinese barbecue sauce, it is made with fermented mashed soybeans, salt, sugar, and garlic.
Kumquat:	Tiny oval-shaped, yellow-orange citrus fruit.
Longan:	Small and round with a smooth, brown skin and clear pulp, it comes in clusters when fresh, but the canned product is more common.
Loquats:	Smooth, yellow-orange fruit.
Lotus root:	Tuberous stem of the water lily.
Lychee:	Also spelled lichee or litchi; a small delicate, juicy, round fruit.
Mock duck:	Vegetarian mixed dish that commonly consists of wheat gluten cooked with vegetables.
Pomelo:	Also known as Chinese grapefruit, this citrus fruit is green, yellow, or pink in color.
Rice, glutinous:	Also known as sweet or sticky rice, it is a short-grained, opaque, pearl white rice that becomes sticky when cooked.

Rice vermicelli: Thin, white noodles made from rice flour, they are often used as an alternative to rice.

Spring roll wrapper: Thin sheets, larger than wonton wrappers, made from rice flour.

Taro: Starchy, tuberous, rough-textured brown root.

Wonton: A steamed or fried wrapper filled with minced pork and/or shrimp.

Wonton wrappers: Thin, yellow sheets made of flour, egg, salt, and water.

Yard-long beans: Grown to a length of up to 18 inches, they are thinner and more flexible than snap beans and very tender.

SAMPLE MENU

▲ Chinese ▲

Menu	Exchanges
Wonton Soup (one cup)	1 starch/bread, 1 fat
Chicken Moo Goo Gai Pan (two cups)	1 starch/bread, 2 lean meat 1 to 2 vegetable
Steamed rice (⅔ cup)	2 starch/bread
Fortune cookie (one)	1 fruit
Total:	4 starch/bread 2 lean meat 1 to 2 vegetable 1 fruit 1 fat
Calories:	600
Carbohydrate:	85 gm (58%)
Protein:	30 gm (20%)
Fat:	15 gm (22%)

If your meal plan does not include all these exchanges, you must make some decisions. See Chapter 30 for guidelines.

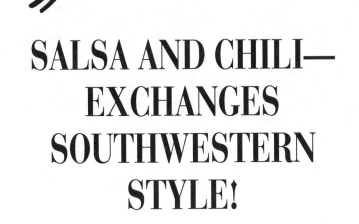

SALSA AND CHILI—
EXCHANGES
SOUTHWESTERN
STYLE!

The American Southwest—in movies it's the land of the permanent sunset...romantic, exotic, exciting. The Southwest reveals a unique blending of several backgrounds—Mexican, American Indian, Spanish, and American pioneer cultures, and a cuisine that is a delicious melding of distinctive and appealing flavors. Southwest cuisine is more than just chilies, corn, and beans served Tex/Mex style. To add spice and variety to your eating, try some of the dishes influenced by our neighbors to the south and west.

Beans are a staple food and are found in many dishes and combinations. Refried beans are commonly made from pinto beans and are frequently eaten. Kidney and black beans are also found in Indian and Mexican cuisine.

Tortillas, another staple that echoes Mexican influence, come in two versions: the slightly coarse light, golden cornmeal variety and softer flour tortillas made with white flour. Soft tortillas contain little fat; taco shells are deep-fried. When served with a meal, tortillas should be served warm.

Today, the chili is one of the world's most popular spices. More than 100 varieties are grown and, in general, the smaller the pepper, the hotter; the larger the pepper, the milder. Salsa (a red tomato sauce) is used as the "salt and pepper" of the Southwest. Depending upon the chilies used, flavor ranges from mild to fiery hot.

Meats are frequently grilled over mesquite fires. Mesquite is a type of wood from a Southwestern tree or shrub, giving a distinctive flavor to meats. Chicken and beef are frequently used along with eggs and potatoes.

Be aware that lard, salt pork, bacon fat, or other animal fat drippings are frequently used in Mexican cooking. When preparing Mexican foods yourself, make appropriate substitutions for these saturated fats. Lean-beef-, chicken-, or bean-filled soft burritos, enchiladas, and tacos are excellent choices. Top with extra salsa or salsa verde (green chili sauce) or sauces made from low-fat or plain yogurt. Go easy on the use of sour cream, guacamole, and grated cheese.

For an appetizer, try a gazpacho soup, seviche (marinated seafood), or a salad of mixed greens, tomato, and onion. Shrimp or fish Veracruz (with tomato sauce), arroz con pollo (chicken with rice—remove skin), chicken, beef or shrimp fajitas; along with soft chicken tacos; soft bean, vegetable, or fish burritos; chicken, seafood, or bean enchiladas with green chili sauce or hot sauce are other good choices.

It's interesting to note that the only beverage able to hold its own against the hottest chili peppers is tequila. Tequila, not necessarily recommended, however, is alcohol distilled from the fermented juice of the maguey cactus plant, which thrives in the Mexican state of Jalisco.

▲ EXPANDED EXCHANGES ▲

Southwestern/Mexican Cooking

FOOD	QUANTITY	EXCHANGES
Starch/Bread:		
Breadfruit	2 pieces, 2" x 1" wedge	1 starch/bread
Cassava	½ cup	1 starch/bread
Corn, taco, or tortilla chips	1 cup (1 oz.)	1 starch/bread 2 fat
Dahl	½ cup	1 starch/bread
Frijoles cocidos	⅓ cup	1 starch/bread
Frijoles cocidos	1 cup	2 starch/bread 1 lean meat
Frijoles refritoes (refried beans)	⅓ cup	1 starch/bread 1 fat
Hard roll, 3"	1	1 starch/bread
Hard roll, 6"	⅓	1 starch/bread
Hominy	½ cup	1 starch/bread
"Hops" bread	1 small	1 starch/bread
Jicama	1 cup	1 starch/bread
Malanga	⅓ cup	1 starch/bread
Masa harina	2 tablespoons	1 starch/bread
Plantain, mature, cooked	⅓	1 starch/bread
Spanish rice	⅓ cup	1 starch/bread 1 fat

FOOD	QUANTITY	EXCHANGES
Taco shell, 6" diameter	2	1 starch/bread 1 fat
Tortillas		
Corn, 6"	1	1 starch/bread
Flour, 8"	1	1 starch/bread
Flour, 12"	½	1 starch/bread
Vermicelli	½ cup	1 starch/bread
Yam, white	⅓ cup	1 starch/bread
Yautia	1 small **or** ⅓ cup boiled	1 starch/bread
Lean Meat:		
Menudo (tripe soup)	½ cup	1 lean meat
Skirt steak	1 oz.	1 lean meat
Medium Fat Meat:		
Queso Fresco	1 oz.	1 med. fat meat
Queso Mexican	1 oz.	1 med. fat meat
Queso "Jalisco"	1 oz.	1 med. fat meat
Goat	4 small cubes	1 med. fat meat
High Fat Meat:		
Chorizo, beef or pork	1 oz.	1 high fat meat 1 fat
Vegetable:		
Amaranth, cooked	½ cup	1 vegetable
Calabazita, Mexican squash, cooked	½ cup	1 vegetable
Chayote (squash)	½ cup	1 vegetable
Cactus leaves (nopales)	½ cup	1 vegetable
Hot chili peppers (jalapeno)	4 peppers	1 vegetable
Ensalada de aquacite, (sliced avocado with tomato and lettuce)	½ cup	1 vegetable 3 fat
Gazpacho	½ cup	1 vegetable 1 fat
Jicama	½ cup	1 vegetable
Okra	½ cup	1 vegetable
Tomatoes, small green	½ cup **or** 2	1 vegetable
Verdolages (purslane)	½ cup	1 vegetable

FOOD	QUANTITY	EXCHANGES
Fruit:		
Cherimoya	½ small	1 fruit
Guava	½	1 fruit
Apple banana	½ medium	1 fruit
Cactus fruit	1 medium	1 fruit
Coco plum	1 medium	1 fruit
Mamey	½ medium	1 fruit
Mango	½ small	1 fruit
Guava nectar	½ cup	1 fruit
Papaya	1 cup	1 fruit
Sapota (custard apple)	1 small	1 fruit
Spanish sauce	½ cup	1 fruit
Fat:		
Ackee	3 pieces	1 fat
Avocado, 4" diameter	⅛	1 fat
Ghee	1 teaspoon	1 fat
Guacamole	2 tablespoons	1 fat
Sofrito	2 teaspoons	1 fat
Free Foods:		
Chilies		
Chili salsa		
Cilantro, fresh		
Taco sauce		
Combination Foods:		
Beef Cubes in Brown Gravy (carne guisada)	1 cup	1 starch/bread 2 med. fat meat 1 fat
Burrito de Carne (meat with flour tortilla) (If deep-fried add extra fat)	1 small, 7" tortilla	2 starch/bread 2 med. fat meat 1 fat
	1 large, 9" tortilla	3 starch/bread 3 med. fat meat 1 fat
Burrito de Frijoles Refritos (beans with flour tortilla) (If deep-fried add 1 to 2 extra fats)	1 small, 7"	3 starch/bread 1 med. fat meat 1 fat
	1 large, 9"	4 starch/bread 1½ med. fat meat 2 fat

FOOD	QUANTITY	EXCHANGES
Chili con Carne without beans	1 cup	½ starch/bread 3 med. fat meat
Chili con Carne with Beans	1 cup	2 starch/bread 2 med. fat meat
Chili Rellenos	7"	2 starch/bread 2 med. fat meat 1 vegetable 2 fat
Chili Verde (diced meat, green chili, rice or beans)	1 cup	1 starch/bread 3 med. fat meat 1 vegetable 2 fat
Chimichangas, all varieties	1 (6 oz.)	3 starch/bread 2 med. fat meat 2 fat
Corn Fritters	1 serving	1 starch/bread 2 med. fat meat 1 fat
Enchiladas, Beef (6" tortilla, ground beef, mozzarella cheese, red chili sauce)	1	2 starch/bread 2 med. fat meat 1 fat
Enchiladas, Cheese (6" tortilla, mozzarella cheese, red chili sauce)	1	2 starch/bread 1 to 2 med. fat meat 2 fat
Enchirito with Cheese, Beef, and Beans	1	2 starch/bread 2 med. fat meat 1 fat
Flauta (rolled, filled fried corn tortilla)	1	1 starch/bread 1 med. fat meat
Frijoles with Cheese	1 cup	2 starch/bread 1 med. fat meat 2 fat
Mexican or Spanish Rice (rice, tomato sauce, green chilies)	½ cup	1 starch/bread 1 vegetable 1 fat
Nachos with Cheese	6–8 nachos	2½ starch/bread 1 high fat meat 1 fat

FOOD	QUANTITY	EXCHANGES
Nachos with Cheese, Beans, Ground Beef	6–8 nachos	3½ starch/bread 2 med. fat meat 3 fat
Picadillo	¾ cup	1 starch/bread 2 med. fat meat 2 fat
Quesadillas (6" corn or 7" flour tortilla, green chilis, mozzarella cheese)	1	1 starch/bread 2 med. fat meat 2 fat
Rice with Chicken (arroz con pollo)	¾ cup	1 starch/bread 2 med. fat meat 1 fat
Mexican Squash with Beef (calabazita con carne)	½ cup	1 med. fat meat 1 vegetable 1 fat
Yellow Squash and Chicken	¾ cup	2 lean meat 1 vegetable 2 fat
Open Taco (tortilla, ground beef, lettuce, chili sauce)	1	1 starch/bread 3 med. fat meat 1 vegetable
Taco (7" tortilla, meat. cheese, tomato, lettuce)	1	1 starch/bread 1 to 2 med. fat meat 1 fat
Taco	1 large	3 starch/bread 3 med. fat meat 3 fat
Taco Salad	1½ cups	1½ starch/bread 1½ med. fat meat 1 fat
Beef Tamales with Sauce	2 small **or** 1 large	2 starch/bread 1 to 2 med. fat meat 2 fat
Tostada or Tortilla with Refried Beans	1 small	2 starch/bread 2 fat
Tostada with Beef	1 small	1 starch/bread 1 med. fat meat 1 fat

FOOD	QUANTITY	EXCHANGES
Tostada with Beans, Beef and Cheese	1 large	2 starch/bread 2 med. fat meat 2 fat
Tostada with Beef and Cheese	1 large	1½ starch/bread 2 med. fat meat 1 fat
Tostada with Guacamole	1 large	2 starch/bread 1 med. fat meat 3 fat
Vermicelli or Rice with Beef (fidelio con carne)	1 cup	2 starch/bread 2 med. fat meat 1 fat

Word List

Arroz: Rice.

Arroz con pollo: Rice with chicken, tomatoes, and spices.

Burrito: A soft flour tortilla filled with beans, ground beef, chicken, or cheese. It is rolled and covered with a sauce or deep-fried.

Calabazita:
(Mexican
squash) Similar in size and shape to the cucumber, except the skin is light green. Simmered with onion and spices and often combined with meat in a casserole dish.

Carne: Meat.

Carne guisada: Beef tips sauteed with chopped onions, green pepper, and chili peppers. Stewed tomatoes are added and the combination is simmered until tender.

Cassava
(Yucca root): Starchy root, also called "manioc." It has a bitter odor that disappears after cooking. It is not eaten raw.

Chayote: Mexican squash that is green, pear-shaped, and some-times covered with tiny hairs.

Cherimoya: It has a rough green outer skin. When ripened and chilled, the flesh has a sherbet-like texture.

Chili: Refers to the chili pepper, which ranges in flavor from mild to sweet to pungent and red hot. They can be used fresh, canned, or dried or as an ingredient in sauces or dishes.

Chili con carne: Referred to commonly as chili. A hearty meat soup made with tomato, onions, peppers, kidney beans, spices, and beef.

Chili powder: Blend of chili, herbs, and spices.

Chili rellenos: Green chili pepper filled with cheese and wrapped in a rich egg batter. Deep-fried and smothered in chili verde.

Chimichanga: Flour tortilla filled and folded like a burrito, then deep-fried.

Chorizo: A highly seasoned sausage of chopped beef or pork with sweet red peppers. The preparation is fried and eaten in a taco, burrito, or tortilla mixed with scrambled eggs or eaten as an entree.

Cilantro: The fresh leaves and stems of the coriander plant, it imparts a distinctive flavor to salsa, meat dishes, and soups.

Enchilada: Oil-blanched corn tortilla folded (or rolled) around a filling of beef or cheese. It can be covered with a sauce of chili con carne, tomato, cheese, or guacamole and garnished with chopped onions and grated cheese.

Enchirito: Enchilada with meat, chilies, beans, and sauce.

Fajitas: Sauteed onions, peppers, tomatoes, choice of chicken, beef, or shrimp, sauteed with Mexican spices. Served in skillet with flour tortillas and salsa on side.

Fidelio con carne: Sauteed beef cubes combined with browned vermicelli, tomatoes, and spices.

Frijoles: Beans are served in some form at every meal in Mexico. They are simmered until tender with onion, cilantro, chili pepper, diced tomatoes, and seasonings.

Frijoles cocidos: Beans that are boiled.

Frijoles refritos: Popularly known as refried beans. Beans are simmered with bacon, onion, garlic, whole tomatoes, cilantro, and herbs until soft. Then they are mashed and fried slowly. Chili powder may be added.

Guacamole: Mashed avocado mixture. Sometimes seasoned with salsa, chopped chili and other seasonings.

Guava: A sweet juicy fruit ranging in color from green to yellow with red or yellow flesh.

Harina: Flour.

Jicama: A tan, turnip-like vegetable whose crisp, white flesh is juicy. Delicious in a salad or served raw and cold, plain or with a sprinkling of lime.

Maiz: Corn, maize.

Malanga: Large herb with starchy, thick, tuberous, white edible root.

Manteca: Lard.

Masa harina: Specially-prepared corn flour used to make corn tortillas, tamales, and nachos.

Menudo: Soup of tripe and hominy.

Nachos: Fried tortilla chips with cheese.

Nopales (cactus): The leaves or pods of the prickly pear cactus are sliced in strips and cooked with onions and spices. They taste like crisp green beans.

Picante: The Mexican word for hot and spicy.

Plantain: Greenish looking banana with rough skin and a number of blemishes. It is used as a vegetable rather than a fruit because the fruit remains starchy, even when fully ripe. Never eaten raw.

Quesadillas: Tortillas filled with cheese and heated or fried until cheese melts. They are eaten with salsa, usually as snacks.

Queso fresco, Blanco, or Mexicano: White, crumbly Mexican cheese which is low in fat. Similar to cottage cheese.

Salsa: A combination of tomato, chilies, and onions used as the salt and pepper of the Southwest. Depending upon the chilies used, flavor ranges from mild to fiery hot.

Sapota: Also called the Mexican custard apple. Clusters of the fruit are large, greenish-yellow. They resemble green apples in appearance.

Spanish rice: White rice sauteed in a skillet with tomatoes, green peppers, onions, and seasonings.

Taco: A crisp, deep-fried corn tortilla folded in half to hold seasoned ground beef, diced tomatoes, shredded lettuce, and cheese.

Tamarind: The fruit is a long, flattened pod, cinnamon brown in color.

Tortilla: Baked, flat, round thin cakes of unleavened cornmeal (masa) or wheat flour. The bread of Mexico.

Tamales: Extruded cooked corn masa wrapped around a chili beef filling. A sauce of chili con carne, tomato, or cheese can be used as an accompaniment.

Tostadas: Tortillas that have been fried until golden brown and crisp in hot lard or oil. They are then served with various combinations of meat, poultry, sauces, chilies, lettuce, and tomatoes.

Verdolagas: Purslane; leaves that can be eaten in a salad; tender leaves and young stalks can also be cooked like spinach.

Yautia: A starchy edible tuber that is cooked and eaten like yams or potatoes.

SAMPLE MENU

▲ Mexican ▲

Menu	Exchanges
Chicken Enchilada	2 starch/bread
(one)	2 med. fat meat
	1 fat
Beef Taco	1 starch/bread
(one)	1 med. fat meat
	1 fat
Refried Beans	1 starch/bread
(⅓ cup)	1 fat
Spanish Rice	1 starch/bread
(⅓ cup)	1 fat
Total:	5 starch/bread
	3 med. fat meat
	4 fat
Calories:	800
Carbohydrate:	75 gm (38%)
Protein:	35 gm (18%)
Fat:	40 gm (44%)

With a Mexican menu, chances are good you will need to make decisions. You can also see why it will be important to be careful of fat choices at other times during the day! Choose what to eat, what to take home in a "doggie bag," or what to leave if everything does not fit into your meal plan.

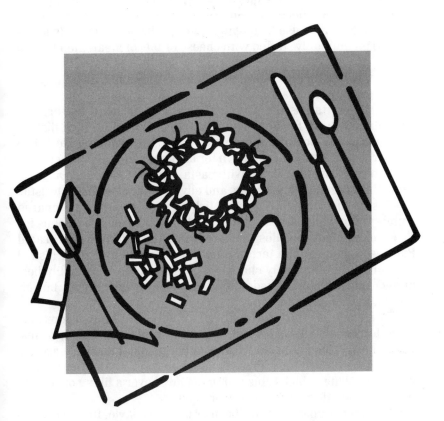

PASTA, PARMIGIANA, PRIMAVERA—EXCHANGES ITALIANO

One of the most enjoyable aspects of Italian cooking is its diversity, which reflects the country's varied geography and climate. Pasta is a common dish throughout Italy. In the north, pasta (such as ravioli) is commonly stuffed with cheese or bits of meat, then topped with a cream sauce, whereas in the south it is usually served unfilled, with a tomato sauce. Seasonings common to all of Italy are garlic, parsley, and basil.

Northern Italy is the principal producer of meat, butter, and cheese, and these foods are a major part of the diet. Rice dishes, such as risotto, polenta, a cornmeal mush, are widely eaten. The area around Genoa is best known for its pesto sauce, a basil, cheese, and nut paste usually served with pasta. Lighter foods, such as fresh vegetables prepared with herbs and olive oil, are also characteristic.

Just to the south, in Tuscany, fish and vegetables are prepared simply using wine, olive oil and fresh herbs. Florence is famous for its green spinach noodles that are served with butter and grated Parmesan cheese. The term *Florentine* refers to a dish garnished with or containing finely chopped spinach. Rome is probably best known for fettucine Alfredo, long egg noodles mixed with butter, cream, and grated cheese.

The regions south of Rome, like Sicily, are known for their "Mediterranean" diet of low-fat, low cholesterol foods. Pasta, grains, vegetables, dried beans, and fish—with little meat and oil— are the cuisine of southern Italy. Pizza is native to Naples. Another form of pizza is calzone, which is pizza dough folded over a filling of cheese, ham, and/or salami, then baked or fried.

Whether prepared in southern or northern style, Italian cuisine has become one of our most popular ethnic cuisines and a part of American culture. The various cuisines blend together and when appropriate choices are made can add up to much good healthful eating in Italian restaurants or delicatessens.

If you order a pasta dish, avoid the cream and cheese sauces. Better choices are pastas with tomato sauce (such as marinara), vegetable sauce (such as primavera), white wine sauce, or lemon butter sauce (piccata). Although olive oil is popular, remember that it contains 120 calories per tablespoon, so ask to limit the amount used.

Italian meals begin with the *antipasto*, which means "before the food." This is followed by the *primi* or first course, which is usually pasta, but may be soup or rice. Next is the second course or *secondi*, which is the fish, chicken, veal, or other meat-type item. This course is usually served with a vegetable. A salad, *insalata*, follows the meal.

Begin your meal with one of the following choices: zuppa de pesce (fish soup), minestrone, chicken broth with pasta, steamed clams or mussels marinara, marinated artichokes, roasted pepper salad, tomato and onion salad, focaccia (a flat round bread), or bruschetta (garlic toast with a small amount of olive oil). Continue with one of the following: risotto (without butter), pasta with tomato and basil, pasta with marinara sauce, chicken ravioli with marinara sauce, pasta primavera, linguini with red clam sauce, polenta (without butter or cheese), chicken cacciatore, cioppino (an elaborate fish stew), broiled fish with tomato-based sauce, or chicken marsala. Finish your meal with an Italian ice or fresh fruit and an espresso or cappuccino.

Let's look at how some of these Italian choices can be incorporated into an exchange meal plan.

▲ EXPANDED EXCHANGES ▲

Italian Cooking

FOOD	QUANTITY	EXCHANGES
Starch/Bread:		
Alfredo sauce	½ cup	1½ starch/bread
		1 med. fat meat
		1 fat
Bolognese sauce	½ cup	1 starch/bread
		1 fat
Gazpacho	1½ cup	1 starch/bread
Gnocchi dumplings	2 small	1 starch/bread
Italian bread	1 slice (1 oz.)	1 starch/bread
Italian bread with garlic butter	1 slice (1 oz.)	1 starch/bread
		1–2 fat

FOOD	QUANTITY	EXCHANGES
Marinara sauce	½ cup	1 starch/bread 1 fat
Meat flavor or mushroom spaghetti sauce	½ cup	1 starch/bread 1 fat
Minestrone soup	1 cup	1 starch/bread 1 fat
Pastas	½ cup	1 starch/bread
Red clam sauce	1 cup	1 starch/bread 1 fat
Spaghetti sauce	½ cup	1 starch/bread 1 fat
Spaghetti sauce with meat	½ cup	1 starch/bread 1 med. fat meat
Vermicelli soup	1 cup	1 starch/bread
Medium Fat Meat:		
Prosciutto (Italian ham)	1 oz.	1 med. fat meat
Meatballs	1, 2" diameter	1 med. fat meat
High Fat Meat:		
White clam sauce	½ cup	1 high fat meat
Vegetable:		
Gazpacho	½ cup	1 vegetable
Italian green beans	½ cup	1 vegetable
Pizza sauce	¼ cup	1 vegetable
Ratatouille	½ cup	1 vegetable 1 fat
Tomato paste	1 tablespoon	1 vegetable
Tomato puree	¼ cup	1 vegetable
Tomato sauce	⅓ cup	1 vegetable
Fats:		
Alfredo sauce	2 tablespoons (1 oz.)	2 fat
Pesto sauce	2 tablespoons (1 oz.)	3 fat
Combination Dishes:		
Cannelloni	4 stuffed noodles	2 starch/bread 3 med. fat meat 2 fat

FOOD	QUANTITY	EXCHANGES
Cannelloni Florentine (veal, spinach, and beef)	4 stuffed noodles	2 starch/bread 2 med. fat meat 2 fat
Chicken Cacciatore with sauce	chicken breast	1 starch/bread 3 lean meat 1 vegetable
Chicken Parmigian with Noodles	chicken breast, ½ cup noodles	1 starch/bread 1 vegetable 3 lean meat 1 fat
Chicken or Turkey Tetrazzini (pollo alla tetrazzini)	1 cup	2 starch/bread 1 vegetable 2 med. fat meat
Eggplant Parmigiana	1 cup	1 starch/bread 1 vegetable 2 med. fat meat 1 fat
Fettuccini Primavera	1½ cup	2 starch/bread 1 vegetable 1 med. fat meat 2 fat
Fettuccini with Chicken	1 cup	2 starch/bread 2 med. fat meat 1 fat
Spaghetti with Meat Sauce	1 cup	2 starch/bread 1 vegetable 1 med. fat meat
Spaghetti with Meatballs (spaghetti con polpette)	1 cup (with 6 small meatballs	2 starch/bread 1 vegetable 2 med. fat meat
Spaghetti with Tomato Sauce	1 cup	3 starch/bread 1 vegetable
Lasagna (3" x 4")	1 serving	1 starch/bread 2 med. fat meat 1 vegetable
Linguini with White Clam Sauce	1 cup	3 starch/bread 2 med. fat meat 1 fat

FOOD	QUANTITY	EXCHANGES
Manicotti with Ricotta Cheese and Tomato Sauce	2 shells	2 starch/bread 2 med. fat meat 1 fat
Pizza with Cheese, Sausage, Pepperoni pizza	¼ of a 16 to 18 oz.	2 starch/bread 2 med. fat meat 1 vegetable 1 fat
Ravioli with Beef	1 cup	2 starch/bread 1 med. fat meat 1 vegetable
Ravioli with Cheese	1 cup	2 starch/bread 1 med. fat meat 1 vegetable 2 fat
Veal Marsala	1 cutlet	1 vegetable 3 med. fat meat
Veal Parmigiana	1 cutlet	2 starch/bread 3 med. fat meat 1 vegetable 1 fat

Word List

Antipasto:	Appetizers.
Cannelloni:	Hollow pasta that is filled with ricotta cheese, meat, and/or spinach and served with cheese and tomato sauce.
Chicken cacciatore:	Sauteed chicken pieces simmered in a meatless tomato sauce.
Fettucini Alfredo:	Thin, flat pasta served with a creamy cheese sauce.
Florentine:	A dish garnished with or containing finely ground spinach.
Fusilli primavera:	Spiral, long pasta topped with sauteed vegetables.

Gnocchi: Little dumplings, made from white flour, potato, or a combination of both; often topped with sauce.

Italian green beans (Romano): Wide, quick-cooking green beans that are often served in a sauce.

Lasagna: Very wide, flat pasta served with meat, cheese, and tomato sauce.

Manicotti: Large tubular pasta served with a filling of meat or cheese and with meatless tomato sauce.

Pasta: Includes fettuccine, linguine, spaghetti, cannelloni, macaroni, elbow, shells, noodles, rigatoni, rotelle, vermicelli, etc.

Pesce: Seafood.

Pesto: A basil, cheese, and nut paste usually served with pasta.

Polenta: Cornmeal and water mixture, baked and served with a sauce.

Pollo: Chicken.

Ravioli: A pasta square stuffed with eggs, vegetables, cheese, or meat and covered with tomato sauce.

Risotto: Italian short-grain rice that has a creamy consistency when cooked; often mixed with butter and cheese before serving.

Veal parmigiana: Thin slices of veal, pounded for tenderness, rolled in bread crumbs, and Parmesan cheese, covered with mozzarella cheese and a meatless tomato sauce.

White clam sauce: White-wine-based cream sauce containing whole clams.

Zuppe: Soup.

SAMPLE MENU

▲ Italian ▲

Menu	Exchanges
Minestrone	1 starch/bread
	1 fat
Italian Bread with Garlic Butter	1 starch/bread
	2 fat
Veal Cacciatore (veal cutlet	3 med. fat meat
served with spaghetti and topped	3 starch/bread
with marinara sauce)	1 fat
Insalata di Casa (house salad	1 vegetable
greens, tomato, onion) with	
Italian Dressing	1 fat
Italian Ice	1 fruit or starch/bread

Total:	5 starch/bread
	3 med. fat meat
	1 vegetable
	1 fruit
	5 fat

Calories:	950
Carbohydrate:	95 gm. (41%)
Protein:	40 gm. (16%)
Fat:	45 gm. (43%)

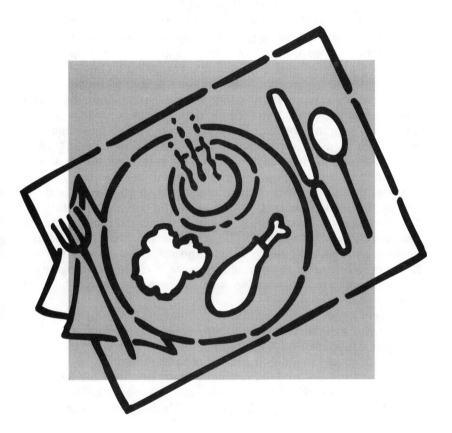

KEEPING KOSHER—
EXCHANGES FOR
JEWISH COOKERY

"**K**osher," defined as "proper" or "fit" or "in accordance with religious law," is used to describe the specific dietary and lifestyle guidelines sanctioned by Jewish law. It relates to aspects of what, when, where, and how one eats and lives. For example, kosher laws dictate method of slaughter preparation and service of meat, as well as the way various meals are prepared and served. In kosher households, meat and dairy meals are separated; the dishes and utensils are also separated for meat and dairy meals. This is known as "keeping kosher." The word "traif," which describes animals found non-kosher because of physical damage or imperfections, is commonly used to describe all foods that are non-kosher.

The traditional eating patterns of Jewish people are based on the laws of Kashrut, which are the general dietary laws from the Torah, the Jewish book of written laws and their interpretations. The Torah encompasses the five books of Moses and the customs for celebrating Jewish holidays. These laws are observed in varying degrees by orthodox, conservative, and reformed denominations. In general, orthodox Jews would be more likely to observe Jewish dietary laws than conservative Jews. Reform Jews would be least likely to follow them.

A very important aspect of planning meals according to the laws of Kashrut is the forbiddance of mixing meat (fleischig) or poultry with dairy foods (milchig). Dairy and meat or poultry products may not be eaten at the same meal. After eating meat, kosher households must wait one to six hours before dairy products can be eaten. However, dairy products may be eaten before the meat. Meat foods may then be eaten after rinsing the mouth and a brief wait—often one-half or one hour.

Meats that come from animals that chew their cud, have split hooves (cattle, sheep, goats, and deer), and have been slaughtered in a kosher manner and have had the additional step of being koshered through a soaking and salting process are acceptable. Pig and pork products are not kosher, nor are birds of prey. Chicken, turkey, goose, pheasant, and duck are kosher. Only eggs from kosher birds are allowed.

Fish are considered "pareve" or neutral (categorized as neither meat nor milk). Fish that have both fins and scales are considered kosher and do not require a ritual slaughtering and additional koshering.

All foods that are considered pareve may be served at either meat or dairy meals. All fruits, vegetables, and starches are pareve and considered kosher. Pareve foods contain neither meat nor milk and are prepared in utensils used for pareve only. Many breads, cakes, and cereals are kosher. They are neutral foods if milk, butter, or other dairy products or derivatives are not used.

Many food companies prepare food products that are kosher certified. This is usually indicated on the labels with a ⓤ which represents the Union of Orthodox Jewish Congregations of America (UOJCA). This is a national kosher certification program, operated in conjunction with the Rabbinical Council of America, and certifies more than 15,000 products. The letter "K" may also be used to denote kosher foods.

Bagels (water rolls), rye and pumpernickel breads, and whole grains such as oatmeal, barley, brown rice, and kasha (buckwheat groats) are eaten frequently. Soups, especially chicken noodle, chicken rice, and borscht (hot or cold beet soup), are popular. Spinach or sorrel leaves are used for schav, another popular soup. Broccoli, carrots, sweet potatoes and yams, and cabbage are used extensively. Other traditional dishes use potatoes or noodles, such as kugel (potato or noodle casserole). Cooked or dried fruits are commonly served and stewed fruits may be eaten as desserts with the meat meal.

Historically, the kosher diet has been high in fat. Many cuts of kosher meat are well-marbled with fat. Schmaltz (chicken fat) is a favorite ingredient in many traditional Jewish dishes, used for flavor and even as an ingredient for sandwiches. Fried dishes like blintzes (crepes) and matzo brie (fried matzo) also are popular in kosher cooking. However, in place of schmaltz or butter, small amounts of margarine or kosher certified vegetable oil, which are pareve (neutral and do not contain milk or nonfat dry milk solids), can be used.

Many traditional dishes are also high in sodium. The koshering process is a salting process, and kosher meats and poultry tend to be high in sodium. Fresh kosher fish does not have to be salted to be kosher. In preparing your own dishes, you can use substitutes for high saturated fat and high salt products.

▲ EXPANDED EXCHANGES ▲

Jewish Cooking

FOOD	QUANTITY	EXCHANGES
Bread/Starches:		
Bagel	½	1 starch/bread
Bialy (roll)	½ (1 oz.)	1 starch/bread
Bulke (roll)	½ medium	1 starch/bread
Challah (hallah)	1 slice (1 oz.)	1 starch/bread
Farfel, dry	3 tablespoons	1 starch/bread
Hard roll	½	1 starch/bread
Kasha (buckwheat groats)		
cooked	½ cup	1 starch/bread
dry	2 tablespoons	1 starch/bread
Kichlach	3, 1"square	1 starch/bread
Lentils	⅓ cup	1 starch/bread
Lokshen (noodles)	½ cup	1 starch/bread
Matzo	6" (¾ oz.)	1 starch/bread
Matzo balls (knaidlach)	1 (1½ oz.)	1 starch/bread 1 fat
Matzo crackers	1½" **or** 7	1 starch/bread
Matzo kugel	½ serving	1 starch/bread 1 fat
Matzo meal	2½ tablespoons	1 starch/bread
Matzo meal pancakes	1 medium	1 starch/bread 2 fat
Potato knish	3" round **or** 2	1 starch/bread 2 fat
Potato kugel	½ cup	1 starch/bread 1 fat
Potato latkes (potato pancakes)	½ cup raw batter	1 starch/bread 1 fat
	½ pancake	1 starch/bread 1 fat
Potato starch (flour)	2 tablespoons	1 starch/bread
Pumpernickel bread	1 slice (1 oz.)	1 starch/bread
Rye bread	1 slice (1 oz.)	1 starch/bread

FOOD	QUANTITY	EXCHANGES
Split peas, cooked	⅓ cup	1 starch/bread
Lean Meat:		
Caviar	1 oz.	1 lean meat
Flanken	1 oz.	1 lean meat
Gefilte fish	2 oz.	1 lean meat
Kippered herring	1 oz.	1 lean meat
Lox (smoked salmon)	1 oz.	1 lean meat
Pot cheese	¼ cup	1 lean meat
Pickled herring	1 oz.	1 lean meat
Sardines (canned, drained)	2 medium	1 lean meat
Medium Fat Meat:		
Beef tongue	1 oz.	1 med. fat meat
Brisket	1 oz.	1 med. fat meat
Chopped livers	¼ cup	1 med. fat meat
Corned beef	1 oz.	1 med. fat meat
Sablefish, smoked	1 oz.	1 med. fat meat
Salmon, canned	¼ cup	1 med. fat meat
High Fat Meat:		
Pastrami	1 oz.	1 high fat meat
Stewed chicken	1 oz.	1 high fat meat
Vegetable:		
Borscht (beet soup with sour cream)	½ cup	1 vegetable 1 fat
Sauerkraut	½ cup	1 vegetable
Sorrel (schav)	½ cup	1 vegetable
Fat:		
Chicken fat (schmaltz)	1 teaspoon	1 fat
Cream cheese	1 tablespoon	1 fat
Grebenes (schmaltz cracklings)	1 teaspoon	1 fat
Nondairy creamer, liquid	1 tablespoon	1 fat
Nondairy creamer, powdered	4 teaspoons	1 fat
Sour cream	2 tablespoons	1 fat
Sour cream, lean or light	3 tablespoons	1 fat
Free:		
Horseradish		
Pickles, dill		

FOOD	QUANTITY	EXCHANGES
Combination:		
Cabbage-Beet Borscht	1 cup	1 starch/bread 1 fat
Cheese Blintzes	8 oz. entree	2 starch/bread 2 med. fat meat 3 fat
Chicken and Dumplings	8 oz.	2 starch/bread 2 med. fat meat 3 fat
Cholent with Meat	1 cup	2 starch/bread 1 vegetable 2 med. fat meat 1–2 fat
Cholent, Meatless	1 cup	3 starch/bread 1–2 vegetable 1–2 fat
Kreplach, Meat	2 small	1 starch/bread 2 med. fat meat
Lentil Soup	1 cup	2 starch/bread 1 lean meat
Noodle Pudding	½ cup	2 starch/bread 1 fat
Split Pea Soup	1 cup	2 starch/bread 1 lean meat
Stuffed Cabbage in Tomato Sauce	1 large roll	1 starch/bread 1 vegetable 2 med. fat meat
Sweet Potato Tzimmes	½ cup	1 starch/bread 1 fruit
Tzimmes with Carrots and Apples	½ cup	2 vegetables 1 fruit

These traditional treats, high in sugar and fat, should be avoided:

Bubke (coffeecake)   Lekach (honeycakes)
Hamantaschen (purim tart)   Rugalah (strudel)
Kuchen and Mandel Bread (cake)   Teiglach (pastry)

Word List

Bagel: A hard yeast roll shaped like a doughnut.

Bialy: A flat breakfast roll, softer than a bagel.

Blintzes: Very thin rolled crepe usually filled with cottage or pot cheese or fruit mixture.

Borscht: Soup made with beets, cabbage, or other vegetables. It may be served hot or cold.

Bubke: Coffeecake that is yeast-risen; sweetened with cinnamon and sugar.

Bulke: Large, light yeast roll, softer than a bagel.

Challah: Also spelled hallah. A loaf of very light egg bread, most commonly braided and prepared for the Sabbath and holidays.

Cholent: A slow-cooking stew; can be prepared with or without meat.

Farfel: Noodle dough grated into barley-sized grains and served in soup.

Flanken: Flank steak.

Fleischig: A term describing meat and meat products.

Gefilte fish: A highly seasoned chopped freshwater fish such as carp, pike, or whitefish mixture that is blended with eggs and matzo meal.

Gribenes: Rendered chicken fat and chicken skin fried with onions.

Hamantaschen: Three-cornered cakes made with pastry or cookie crust and filled with poppy seeds, dried fruit, or cheese.

Kasha: Buckwheat groats served as a cooked cereal or as a potato substitute.

Kashrut: A noun describing the Kosher dietary laws based on the Torah.

Kichlach: Light egg cookies.

Kishke: Beef casings stuffed with seasoned filling made from matzo, flour, fat, and onions.

Knaidlach: Matzo balls made of matzo meal, eggs, and fat, generally served in chicken soup.

Knish:	Pastry filled with ground meat, potato, or kasha and spices mixture. The pastry can have a potato base.
Kreplach:	Bite-sized pastry filled with meat or cheese mixture, similar to ravioli.
Kuchen:	Coffeecake.
Kugel:	Pudding or casserole, commonly made with potatoes or noodles.
Latkes:	Pancakes. Potato latkes are very popular.
Leckach:	Honey cake.
Lokshen:	Noodles.
Lox:	Smoked and salted salmon that is cut very thin.
Matzo:	Flat, unleavened cracker.
Matzo meal:	Finely ground matzo used in cooking and baking.
Milchig:	A term describing milk or dairy foods and meals that are dairy.
Pareve:	A term describing neutral foods such as fish, eggs, fruits, and vegetables, which may be served at either a meat or a dairy meal.
Pirogi or piroshkes:	Pastry filled with meat, cheese, or meat stuffing.
Pot cheese:	Cream cheese or other farmer-style cheese.
Schav:	Soup, similar to borscht, made from sorrel.
Schmaltz:	Rendered chicken fat, often used in cooking or pastry making.
Strudel:	Thin pastry rolled up in fruit and nut filling.
Sorrel:	A member of the buckwheat family. Cooked as a green leafy vegetable.
Teiglach:	Small balls of sweet dough cooked in honey.
Traif (Trefe):	Foods that are non-kosher, forbidden, ritually unfit.
Tzimmes:	Versatile, hot side dish often made with dried fruit, carrots, sweet potatoes, and sweetened with honey. Tzimmes may be prepared with meat and served as a main dish or as an accompaniment to a meat meal. Made with fruit only, it is served as a dessert.

SAMPLE MENU

▲ Jewish ▲

Menu	Meal Plan
Challah	1 starch/bread
(one slice)	
Gefilte fish	1 lean meat
(one ounce)	
Horseradish	Free
Beet Borscht	2 vegetables
(one cup)	
Stewed Chicken	3 high fat meat
(3 ounces)	
Potato Kugel	2 starch/bread
(one cup)	2 fat
Fruit Compote	1 fruit
(½ cup)	

Total:	3 starch/bread
	4 meat
	2 vegetable
	1 fruit
	2–3 fat

Calories:	740
Carbohydrate:	70 gm. (38%)
Protein:	40 gm. (22%)
Fat:	35 gm. (40%)

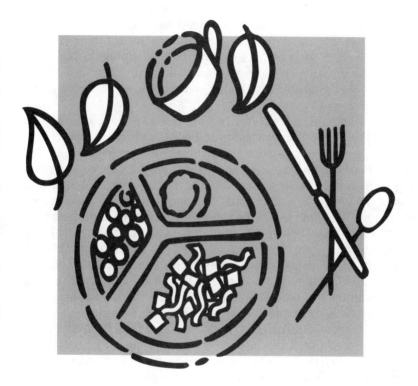

HAPPY TRAILS
TO YOU—
EXCHANGES FOR
CAMPING

Camping is becoming more popular every year because it provides an opportunity to enjoy nature at its very best. Anyone wanting to experience this kind of life should jump into it with enthusiasm. The preparation required will depend on the type of camping you plan to do. When camping with a motor home or camper trailer, you can take nearly any type of food because they are equipped with refrigeration and adequate storage areas for food and cooking utensils. Food for this type of camping will be similar to that eaten at home.

Canoeing and backpacking require more special planning. Food should be compact, lightweight, and nonperishable because it will need to be carried on portages and packed into confined areas of the canoe. For backpacking, everything—including a sleeping bag, cooking equipment, and food—must be carried on your back. For both, space and weight are prime considerations, but the food taken along should be filling and provide a concentrated source of nutrition.

For any type of camping, enough food should be packed for the duration of the trip. Experienced campers solve this problem by planning daily menus. Food for each day can then be packed separately and labeled with the date and time it is to be eaten. The calculated amount of food should be increased slightly to ensure that enough food is available in case a pack is lost or damaged.

Freeze-dried and dried (dehydrated) foods can be used. Freeze-dried foods are best because their flavor is more like fresh foods and they are virtually foolproof in preparation—just add water and serve. When packaged in laminated aluminum foil and vacuum-sealed in plastic, they will last indefinitely if stored in a cool, dry area. Dried foods should be discarded after one year.

Companies that manufacture freeze-dried products, such as AlpineAire and Mountain House will supply nutrition analysis of their products. Addresses for these companies are in the reference section.

Canoers, hikers, or backpackers with insulin-dependent diabetes will need to increase their usual meal plan to allow for the increased activity. In general, begin by increasing calories by 20 percent. On days of very strenuous activities, you may need to eat an extra 1,000 calories a day. Snacks are always important, but even more so with this increased activity. Be sure to plan accordingly.

If milk is not available, or if you do not care for dried skim milk powder, substitute an extra meat, starch, or fruit exchange for your milk exchange.

A camper with diabetes should never assume that fish or berries will be an available food source! Food and all the necessary (and a little extra!) insulin and blood glucose testing supplies should be carefully packed and taken along with you. Medical identification should be worn.

During hard hiking, lunch should be an all-day meal consumed in small, frequent installments to provide a steady flow of fuel without overloading the stomach. Weariness tends to kill the appetite, leading to a vicious cycle of deeper weariness and less appetite!

Insulin dosages may need to be decreased as well. Check with your health care team about how much—it is generally a percentage of your total insulin dose, often beginning with a 10 to 20 percent reduction in your total insulin dosage. Reduce the insulin acting during the time of your activity. For additional guidelines see Chapter 33 on exercise.

▲ EXPANDED EXCHANGES ▲

Camping Foods

FOOD	QUANTITY	EXCHANGES
Starch/Bread:		
Biscuits	2" square, 1	1 starch/bread
		1 fat
Chow mein noodles	½ cup	1 starch/bread
		1 fat
Cooked cereal	½ cup	1 starch/bread
Corn	½ cup rehydrated or 1 oz. dried	1 starch/bread
Cornbread	2" square, 1	1 starch/bread
		1 fat

FOOD	QUANTITY	EXCHANGES
French toast	1 slice	1 starch/bread ½ med. fat meat
Gorp (see recipe in chapter 38)	⅓ cup	1 starch/bread 1 fat
Graham crackers	3 squares	1 starch/bread
Granola (see recipe in chapter 38)	¼ cup	1 starch/bread 1 fat
Granola bar	1 small bar	1 starch/bread 1 fat
Hash browns	½ cup or 2 oz. dried	1 starch/bread 1 fat
Hushpuppies	2" square, 1	1 starch/bread 1 fat
Pancakes	5" diameter, 1	1 starch/bread 1 fat
Pancakes	4" diameter, 3	2 starch/bread 1 fat
Potatoes, mashed	½ cup or 3 oz. dried	1 starch/bread
Potatoes, diced	½ cup or 2 oz. dried	1 starch/bread
Rice, cooked	⅓ cup	1 starch/bread
RyKrisp	4 triple crackers	1 starch/bread
Saltine crackers	6	1 starch/bread
Soup	1 cup	1 starch/bread
Vanilla wafers	6	1 starch/bread
Lean Meat:		
Beef jerky	½ oz.	1 lean meat
Chicken	2 oz. dried	3 lean meat
Chicken, canned	½ 5 oz. can	3 lean meat
Canned shrimp, sardines, etc.	1 oz.	1 lean meat
Dried chipped beef	½ 5 oz. can	3 lean meat
Ham	1 oz.	1 lean meat
Meat sticks	½ oz.	1 lean meat
Tuna fish, canned	½ 7 oz. can	3 lean meat

FOOD	QUANTITY	EXCHANGES
Medium Fat Meat:		
Beef	2 oz. dried	3 med. fat meat
Canned meat	⅛ 2 lb. can	3 med. fat meat
Eggs, prepared	⅓ cup	2 med. fat meat
Pork chops	2 oz. dried	3 med. fat meat
High Fat Meat:		
Cheese	1 oz.	1 high fat meat
Luncheon meat	1 slice (1 oz.)	1 high fat meat
Peanuts	¼ cup (1 oz.)	1 high fat meat
Peanut butter	1 tablespoon	1 high fat meat
Salami	1 slice, ¼"	1 high fat meat
thick (1 oz.)		
Sausage patties	2 oz.	2 high fat meat
Spam	1 slice (3 oz.)	3 high fat meat
Sunflower seeds	¼ cup	1 high fat meat
	(1 oz.)	1 fat
Vegetables:		
Carrots, green	1 oz. dried,	1 vegetable
beans, spinach,	½ cup cooked	
etc.		
Fruit:		
Dried fruit	¼ cup, ½ oz.	1 fruit
Fruit bars	1 bar	1½ fruit
Fruit galaxie	¼ cup	1 fruit
Fruit jerkey	1 strip	1 fruit
Fruit rolls or	1 roll, ½ oz.	1 fruit
roll-ups		
Juice	½ cup	1 fruit
Marshmallows	2 large	1 fruit
Prunes	3	1 fruit
Raisins	2 tablespoons	1 fruit
	(½ oz)	
Stewed fruit	½ cup	1 fruit
Syrup, real maple	¼ cup	4 fruit
	1 tablespoon	1 fruit
Syrup, light	2 tablespoons	1 fruit
Tang or other fruit	½ cup prepared	1 fruit
drinks		

FOOD	QUANTITY	EXCHANGES
Milk:		
Dried nonfat milk powder	⅓ cup powder and ¾ cup water	1 skim milk
Cocoa (see recipe in Chapter 38)	1 cup	1 skim milk
Free:		
Maple syrup made with artificial sweeteners		
Combination Foods:		
Baked Beans and Franks	1 cup	3 starch/bread 1 med. fat meat 1 fat
Beef Stew	1 cup	2 starch/bread 2 med. fat meat 1 to 2 fat
Beef Stroganoff	1 cup	2 starch/bread 2 med. fat meat 1 to 2 fat
Chicken a la King	1 cup	2 starch/bread 2 med. fat meat 1 to 2 fat
Chicken, Beef or Pork Chow Mein (without noodles)	2 cups	1 starch/bread 2 vegetables 2 med. fat meat
Chicken with Dumplings	1½ cups	1 starch/bread 1 vegetable 2 med. fat meat 1 fat
Dumpling	1	1 starch/bread
Chili	1 cup	2 starch/bread 2 med. fat meat 1 fat
Lasagna	1 cup	1 starch/bread 3 med. fat meat 1 to 2 fat
Macaroni and Cheese	1 cup	2 starch/bread 1 med. fat meat 2 fat

FOOD	QUANTITY	EXCHANGES
Spaghetti and Meatballs	1 cup	2 starch/bread 2 med. fat meat 1 to 2 fat
Tuna Noodle Casserole with Peas	1½ cups	2 starch/bread 1 vegetable 2 med. fat meat 1 fat

Desserts:

FOOD	QUANTITY	EXCHANGES
Brownie	2" x 4"	2 starch/bread 2 fat
Cookies	3" diameter	1 starch/bread 1 fat
Cake, white or yellow, no icing	3" square	2 starch/bread 2 fat
Gingerbread	3" x 2"	2 starch/bread 2 fat
Pudding	½ cup	2 starch/bread

SAMPLE MENU

▲ Camping ▲

An example of a typical day's menu would allow for the following type of exchanges at each meal and snack time:

	Menu	Exchanges
Breakfast:	Cooked cereals, biscuits, pancakes, French toast	Starch/bread
	Dried egg powder	Meat
	Fruit juices or dried fruit	Fruit
	Cocoa	Milk
A.M. Snack:	Granola	Starch/bread
Lunch:	RyKrisp	Starch/bread
	Hard salami, cheese, or peanut butter	Meat
	Raisins	Fruit
	Artificially sweetened Kool-Aid	Free
Afternoon Snack:	Graham crackers, RyKrisp, gorp or granola bar	Starch/bread
	Fruit jerkey, raisins, dried fruit	Fruit
	Artificially sweetened Kool Aid	Free
Dinner:	Casseroles using starch/bread and meat exchanges	Starch/bread Meat
	Biscuits or dessert	Starch/bread
	Dried vegetables	Vegetable
	Dried fruit	Fruit
Evening Snack:	Crackers, biscuits, popcorn	Starch/bread
	Cheese, peanuts, sunflower seeds	Meat
	Dried fruit	Fruit
	Dried milk or cocoa	Milk

19

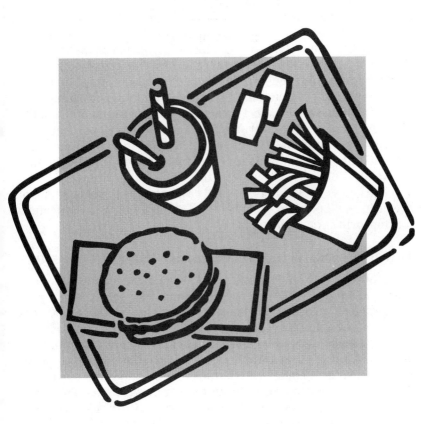

EXCHANGES FOR
THE FAST-FOOD
PHENOMENON

According to a recent survey, more than 133 million people, or more than half the population, eat out or purchase food to go on an average day. The most distinctively American part of this food service business is fast food. Can we still choose fast foods and make choices that are not loaded with grease and calories? The answer, of course, is yes. With careful planning, you can achieve healthful eating.

What kind of sound choices can you make when eating fast-foods? Women should select meals that have between 500 and 600 calories, men between 800 and 900. For women, 30 percent of the calories from fat translates into about 20 to 25 grams per meal. For men, it's about 30 to 35 grams per meal. When figuring sodium intake, the goal is to stay under 1,000 milligrams per meal.

The key to eating at a fast-food restaurant is to know what you are ordering. Let's look at some usual menu items with suggestions for improving your selections.

Burgers—Skip the Mayonnaise-Based Dressings

Scale down to single patties and select basic meat items. For a lower-fat sandwich, have a regular hamburger (or even two plain burgers) instead of a double burger with cheese and special sauces. If you've got a double-decker appetite, pile on lettuce and tomato. Adding cheese adds 100 calories a slice as well as added fat and sodium. While it's true a McDonald's McLean burger is lower in fat, a plain quarter pounder with lettuce and tomato is not such a bad choice either and you can still enjoy a hamburger. What adds extra calories and fat to burgers are the mayonnaise-based dressings. Skip the special sauces on deluxe burgers and you reduce fat and calories.

A big, deluxe hamburger with special sauce, large fries, and a large chocolate chip cookie adds up to 1,200 calories, 64 grams of fat, and 1,385 milligrams of sodium. Compare this with a quarter pounder, regular fries, and diet soda at 630 calories, 43 grams of fat, and 770 milligrams of sodium.

Chicken and Fish—Breading Traps the Fat

Battering, breading, or deep-frying chicken or fish cancels out their normal, low-fat advantages, so if available, choose grilled chicken breasts. If fried is your only choice, choose regular coating over extra crispy varieties (which soak up more oil during cooking) and save as many as 86 calories per piece. Even better, peel off the skin and lose 100 calories, plus most of the fat and excess sodium. Better yet, order mashed potatoes and gravy instead of fries and save 200 calories.

A grilled chicken sandwich has only about 300 to 350 calories and 9 grams of fat. Compare this with deep-fried, breaded chicken sandwiches that generally have 500 to 700 calories and between 30 to 40 grams of fat.

If possible, stick to baked fish. It has half the fat and calories of fried fish and is lower in sodium. Skip the tartar sauce (about 120 calories for 2 tablespoons) and use cocktail sauce (only 35 calories) or lemon juice (zero calories).

Pizza—Extra Toppings, Extra Calories

As a snack or quick meal, pizza can fit nicely into a well-balanced diet. It's not necessarily a low-calorie food, but with its calories it also contributes very respectably to nutrition. Start with thin crust pizza and stay with the regular cheese pizza with mushroom, green pepper, and other vegetable toppings. Two slices of a 16-inch pizza contain 375 calories, only 24 percent of which are from fat. Extra cheese and pepperoni and sausage toppings mean extra fat and calories—as much as 170 calories per slice. By opting for the thin crust over the thick you save up to 130 calories per slice. To avoid extra sodium, skip the olives and anchovies.

Potatoes—Plain Baked Potatoes—A Great Choice

When it comes to potatoes, a plain baked potato is nourishing, filling, and virtually free of fat and sodium. A plain large potato provides 250 calories and 2 grams of fat. Adding cheese sauces, bacon, sour cream, and other toppings can increase the fat level from 2 grams to 30 to 40 grams (5 to 8 teaspoons) and the calories from 250 to 590. A deluxe, superstuffed baked potato with sour cream, butter, bacon, and cheese has 648 calories and 6 teaspoons of fat.

Choose a plain baked potato for lunch or dinner. When combined with a salad and topped with 1/4 cup cottage cheese or one to two tablespoons of grated Swiss, cheddar, or Parmesan cheese, a baked potato becomes a complete meal.

Salads—Complements to Any Fast-Food Meals

A salad bar is a healthful alternative to high-fat sandwiches. Skip the prepared salads (potato, pasta, taco, and so on) and go easy on the dressing. Use of reduced- or low-calorie dressings over regular dressings cuts the calories by at least half. A large salad containing a variety of vegetables, 1/2 cup cottage cheese, and reduced-calorie salad dressing has less than 250 calories. However, by adding just one tablespoon of regular dressing, some bacon bits, and 1/4 cup macaroni or potato salad, you increase the calorie level to 500. A great way to add more fiber to your salad is to add garbanzo beans, those small, round, tan legumes, also known as chickpeas.

Sandwiches—Many Low-Fat Options

If ordering various versions of roast beef, ham, cheese, and turkey sandwiches, your best choices are the regular and junior-sized over the deluxe versions. Skipping the mayonnaise topping (use mustard or horseradish instead) saves at least 100 calories per tablespoon.

Croissant sandwiches are high in calories and fat; one croissant averages 200 to 500 calories. Croissant sandwiches average 400 to 600 calories, which is high compared to 350 calories for the plain roast beef sandwich or 250 calories for a pita sandwich.

Tacos, Tostadas, and Chili—Choices for Adding Fiber

Tacos and tostadas are often good choices. To keep the fat down, skip the sour cream and guacamole and pile on extra salsa and tomatoes.

Chili blows the typical "greasy-spoon" reputation. Even a large bowl of chili has only 300 calories and 12 grams of fat. Beans are one of the best sources of fiber, making chili with beans or baked beans good choices.

Making Healthy Fast-Food Choices

If you do have fast-foods for one meal, try to balance the rest of your day's food choices. A key to making wise choices is to buy small and eat at fast-food restaurants only at mealtime. "Jumbo," "giant," or "deluxe" signal diet caution. Larger serving sizes mean not only additional calories but also more fat, cholesterol, and sodium.

The average calorie count of a fast-food meal is 685, which is not outrageously high. However, many people buy fast-food items as snacks rather than meals. The average calorie count for a so-called snack is 427—more than most people need for a snack!

Choices for a healthy fast-food lunch or dinner may be easier than for breakfast. Start your day with plain muffins, biscuits, or toast. If you order a scrambled egg with an English muffin, you end up with a total of only 366 calories, 17 grams of fat, and 575 milligrams of sodium. Compare this with a sausage and egg biscuit, hash brown potatoes, and large orange juice with 820 calories, 49 grams of fat, and 1,475 milligrams of sodium. Another surprisingly good breakfast option is pancakes without butter.

Studies of fast-food chains show remarkable uniformity in portion sizes and nutritional value of their foods. This means that fast-food chains may be easier to predict than some expensive gourmet restaurants. *Fast Food Facts* can provide you with the nutritional information you need about fast-food items. It's available from many of your favorite bookstores, or see the back of this book for information on how to order.

▲

Guidelines for Choosing Meals at Fast-Food Restaurants

Look for meals that meet the following guidelines:

	Women	Men
Calories, total meal	500–600	800–900
Fat, grams per meal	20–25	30–35
Sodium, milligrams per meal	1,000	1,000

Compare the following choices:

	Calories	Fat (grams)
McLean Deluxe	320	10
or		
Quarter Pounder	410	20
with		
Deluxe Burger	710	44
Grilled Chicken Sandwich	310	9
with		
Deep Fried, Breaded Chicken Sandwich	688	40
or		
Chicken Club Sandwich	621	18
Baked Potato, Plain	250	2
with		
Superstuffed Potato Deluxe	648	38
Pizza, 2 slices Cheese	375	10
with		
Pizza, 2 slices Deluxe	498	20
Chef Salad, reduced-calorie dressing	270	16
with		
Taco Salad	660	37
Soft Serve Cone	144	5
with		
Heath Blizzard	800	24

▲ EXPANDED EXCHANGE LIST ▲

Fast-Food Restaurants

FOOD	QTY.	CALORIES	FAT (gm)	EXCHANGES
Arby's:				
Junior Roast Beef Sandwich	1	218	9	1½ starch/bread 1½ med. fat meat
Regular Roast Beef	1	353	15	2 starch/bread 2 med. fat meat 1 fat
Hot Ham 'n Cheese Sandwich	1	292	14	1 starch/bread 3 med. fat meat
Chicken Breast Sandwich	1	489	26	2 1/2 starch/bread 3 med. fat meat 2 fat
Turkey Deluxe	1	375	17	2 starch/bread 3 med. fat meat
Roasted Chicken	1	254	7	6 lean meat
Tossed Salad with Low-Calorie Italian Dressing	1	57	1	1 vegetable
Baked Potato, Plain	1	290	1	4 starch/bread
Potato Cakes	1	204	12	1½ starch/bread 2 fat
Baskin Robbins:				
Truly Free Frozen Yogurt	½ cup	70	0	1 starch/bread
Frozen Yogurt	⅓ cup	120	1	1 starch/bread
Burger King:				
Hamburger	1	272	11	2 starch/bread 2 med. fat meat
Cheeseburger	1	317	15	2 starch/bread 2 med. fat meat 1 fat
Whopper Jr.	1	322	17	2 starch/bread 2 med. fat meat 1 fat

FOOD	QTY.	CALORIES	FAT (gm)	EXCHANGES
Chicken Tenders with BBQ dipping sauce	6 pieces	275	15	1 starch/bread 2 med. fat meat 1 fat
BK Broiler	1 sandwich	265	8	2 starch/bread 3 lean meat
BK Broiler Sauce	1 order	90	10	2 fat
Garden Salad	1	90	5	1 vegetable 1 fat
Salad Bar without Dressing	1	28	0	1 vegetable
Reduced Calorie Italian Salad Dressing	1 pkg.	30	2	½ fat
French Fries	Regular	235	3	1½ starch/bread 2 fat
Dairy Queen:				
Single Hamburger	1	310	13	2 starch/bread 2 med. fat meat 1 fat
Hot Dog	1	280	16	1½ starch/bread 1 med. fat meat 2 fat
BBQ Beef Sandwich	1	225	4	2 starch/bread 2 lean meat
Grilled Chicken Fillet Sandwich	1	300	8	2 starch/bread 3 lean meat
Fish Sandwich	1	400	17	3 starch/bread 2 med. fat meat 1 fat
French Fries	Small	210	10	2 starch/bread 2 fat
Cone	Regular	230	7	2½ starch/bread 1 fat
DQ Sandwich	1	140	4	1½ starch/bread 1 fat
Dilly Bar	1	210	13	1½ starch/bread 2 fat
Yogurt Cone	Regular	180	<1	2½ starch/bread
Domino's Pizza:				
Cheese Pizza, 16" large	2 slices	376	10	4 starch/bread 2 med. fat meat

FOOD	QTY.	CALORIES	FAT (gm)	EXCHANGES
Ham Pizza, 16" large	2 slices	417	11	4 starch/bread 2 med. fat meat
Hardee's:				
Hamburger	1	260	10	2 starch/bread 1 med. fat meat 1 fat
Roast Beef Sandwich	1	280	11	2 starch/bread 2 med. fat meat 1 fat
Grilled Chicken Breast Sandwich	1	310	10	2 starch/bread 3 lean meat
Side Salad	1	20	1	1 vegetable
Chef Salad	1	214	13	1 vegetable 3 med. fat meat
Bagel	1	200	3	2½ starch/bread
Cool Twist Cone Vanilla, Chocolate	1	180	4	2 starch/bread 1 fat
Kentucky Fried Chicken:				
Original Recipe				
Breast	1	260	15	½ starch/bread 3 med. fat meat
Drumstick	1	152	9	2 med. fat meat
Skinfree Crispy				
Breast	1	296	16	1 starch/bread 3 med. fat meat
Drumstick	1	166	9	2 med. fat meat
Mashed Potatoes with Gravy	1	71	2	1 starch/bread
Corn-on-the-Cob	1	90	2	2 starch/bread
Cole Slaw	1	114	6	2 vegetable 1 fat
Long John Silver's:				
Fish with lemon crumb, baked	3 piece	570	12	5 starch/bread 4 lean meat
Light Portion Fish with lemon crumb, baked, rice and small salad	2 piece	270	5	2 starch/brea 1 vegetable 3 lean meat
Chicken, baked	1 entree	550	15	5 starch/bread 3 med. fat meat

FOOD	QUANTITY	CALORIES	FAT (gm)	EXCHANGES
McDonald's:				
Hamburger	1	255	10	2 starch/bread 1 med. fat meat 1 fat
Quarter Pounder	1	410	21	2 starch/bread 3 med. fat meat 1 fat
McLean Deluxe	1	320	10	2 starch/bread 3 lean meat
McLean Deluxe with Cheese	1	370	14	2 starch/bread 3 lean meat 1 fat
Chicken McNuggets	6 pieces	270	15	1 starch/bread 2 med. fat meat 1 fat
French Fries	medium	320	17	2½ starch/bread 3 fat
Garden Salad	1	50	2	1 vegetable
Chef Salad	1	170	9	1 vegetable 2 med. fat meat
Lite Vinaigrette Dressing	2 oz packet	48	2	1 fat
Egg McMuffin	1	280	11	2 starch/bread 2 med. fat meat
Scrambled Eggs	1	140	10	2 med. fat meat
English Muffin with Butter	1	170	5	2 starch/bread 1 fat
Apple Bran or Blueberry Muffin	1	180	0	2½ starch/bread
Vanilla Lowfat Frozen Yogurt Cone	1	105	1	1½ starch/bread
Pizza Hut:				
Thin-n-Crispy, Cheese, 12" medium pizza	2 slices	398	17	2 starch/bread 1 vegetable 3 med. fat meat
Hand-Tossed Pizza, Pepperoni, 12" medium pizza	2 slices	518	20	4 starch/bread 3½ med. fat meat
Pan Pizza, Cheese, 12" medium pizza	2 slices	492	18	4 starch/bread 3 med. fat meat

FOOD	QTY.	CALORIES	FAT (gm)	EXCHANGES
Rax:				
Roast Beef Sandwich	1 regular	262	10	2 starch/bread 2 med. fat meat
Deluxe Roast Beef	1	498	30	2½ starch/bread 2½ med. fat meat 3 fat
Grilled Chicken Breast Sandwich	1	402		2 starch/bread 3 med. fat meat 2 fat
Gourmet Garden Salad, No Dressing	1 salad	134	6	1 vegetable 1 med. fat meat
Grilled Chicken Garden Salad, No Dressing	1 salad	202	9	1 starch/bread 2 med/fat meat
Lite Italian Dressing	2 oz.	57	3	1 fat
Chocolate Chip Cookie	1 cookie	262	12	2 starch/bread 1 fat
Fat-Free Vanilla Yogurt Shake	1	220	<1	3 starch/bread
Red Lobster:				
Shrimp Cocktail	6 large	90	2	2 lean meat
Sauce	1 oz.	30	0	1 vegetable
Today's Fresh Catch	5 oz.	165	6	4 lean meat
Crab Legs	16 oz.	120	1	4 lean meat
Grilled Chicken Breast	4 oz.	170	6	3 lean meat
Rice Pilaf	4 oz.	140	3	1½ starch/bread 1 fat
Baked Potato	8 oz.	270	trace	3 starch/bread
Broiled Fish Sandwich	4 oz.	300	10	2 starch/bread 3 lean meat
Subway:				
Cold Cut Combo Sub	6"	427	20	3 starch/bread 2 med. fat meat 2 fat
Meatball Sub	6"	459	22	3 starch/bread 2 med. fat meat 2 fat
Turkey Breast Sub	6"	322	10	3 starch/bread 2 med. fat meat
Roast Beef Sub	6"	345	12	3 starch/bread 2 med. fat meat

FOOD	QTY.	CALORIES	FAT (gm)	EXCHANGES
Taco Bell:				
Bean Burrito	1	447	14	4 starch/bread 1 med. fat meat 2 fat
Beef Burrito	1	402	17	2½ starch/bread 2 med. fat meat 1 fat
Tostada	1	243	11	1 starch/bread 2 med. fat meat 1 fat
Taco	1	184	11	1 starch/bread 2 lean meat
Soft Taco	1	213	10	1 starch/bread 1½ med. fat meat 1 fat
Fajita Steak with Guacamole	1	269	13	1 starch/bread 2 med. fat meat 1 fat
Chicken Fajita	1	225	10	1 starch/bread 2 med. fat meat
Wendy's:				
Hamburger, single, plain	1	350	15	2 starch/bread 3 med. fat meat
Grilled Chicken Sandwich	1	290	7	2 starch/bread 3 lean meat
Breaded Chicken Sandwich	1	450	20	3 starch/bread 3 med. fat meat 1 fat
Plain Baked Potato	1	300	<1	4 starch/bread
Sour Cream	1 pkt.	60	6	1 fat
Chili, Large (12 oz.)	1 bowl	290	9	2 starch/bread 3 lean meat
Taco Salad	1	640	30	5 starch/bread 3 med. fat meat 2 fat
Deluxe Garden Salad	1	110	5	2 vegetable 1 fat
Side Salad	1	60	3	1 vegetable 1 fat
Reduced Italian	2 Tbsp.	50	4	1 fat

EXCHANGES FOR
FITTING CONVENIENCE
INTO YOUR MEAL PLAN

In our busy society, we let convenience influence the way we live our lives, particularly our eating habits. If we're not grabbing a bite at a fast-food restaurant, we're looking for a meal that is quick and easy to prepare so we can spend more time on other pursuits.

Convenience foods are the fastest growing processed food group today, because they give us what we demand: quick, easy-to-prepare, good-tasting, and relatively inexpensive meals.

Aside from convenience, consumers care a great deal about other things as well. We are becoming more knowledgeable about nutrition and the effects that different foods have on our health. We want to eat not only to get energy to enjoy our daily activities, but also to ensure good health throughout a long and productive life. The following guidelines can help us meet nutritional goals while enjoying the convenience of convenience foods!

Goal: Limiting Calories to Control Weight

A weight control program that is reasonable in calories as well as nutritionally adequate should provide 1,200 to 1,500 calories a day. Of these calories, about 400 to 500 calories, or a third of the total, should be consumed at dinner. For weight maintenance, many adults' meal plans will be based on an intake of about 1,800 to 2,400 calories, or about 600 to 800 calories at dinner. For help in determining caloric intake, look at the nutritional label or *Convenience Food Facts* to see how many calories are in the food product.

Goal: Reduce Fat Content of Diet

To achieve the goal of 30 percent of your calories from fat, on a weight maintenance intake of 1,800 to 2,400 calories, you should limit fat to 60 to 80 grams per day or 20 to 28 grams of fat per meal. On a weight loss diet of 1,200 to 1,500 calories, fat should be about 40 to 50 grams per day or about 14 to 18 grams of fat per meal.

Use foods that have the number of fat exchanges allowed in your meal plan. (Five grams of fat is equal to one fat exchange or about a teaspoon of fat.) Please remember that you can move fat exchanges from one meal or snack to another. If you know you will need more fat exchanges at dinner, go easy on your fat exchanges earlier in the day.

Goal: Reducing Sodium/Salt Content of Diet

Many convenience foods are high in sodium content. Salt is usually added not to preserve the food, but to satisfy the public's desire for a salty taste. Generally, it's recommended that sodium intake be under 3,000 milligrams per day for the general public and 2,400 milligrams or less per day for people who have been diagnosed as having high blood pressure. At one meal, sodium intake should not exceed 1,000 milligrams; people on sodium-restricted diets should consume less than 700 milligrams per meal. To be labeled low sodium, a food product cannot contain more than 140 milligrams of sodium per serving.

In addition, look for single servings of foods that have less than 400 milligrams of sodium or main meal entrees with less than 800 milligrams of sodium.

Goal: Maintain Your Meal Plan

The charts on the following pages give you average values for several popular convenience foods. For complete information on convenience foods—their calorie, carbohydrate, protein, fat, saturated fat, and sodium amounts—see *Convenience Food Facts. Help for Planning Quick, Healthy, and Convenient Meals* by Arlene Monk, R.D., C.D.E. It's available from many of your favorite bookstores or see the back of this book for information on how to order.

▲

Guidelines for Choosing Convenience Foods

Look for meals that meet these guidelines:

Calories per meal for weight maintenance: 600 to 800

Calories per meal for weight loss: 400 to 500

Fat grams per meal for weight maintenance: 20 to 28

Fat grams per meal for weight loss: 14 to 18

Saturated fat grams per meal: 5 to 7

Cholesterol milligrams per meal: 100

Sodium milligrams per meal: less than 1,000

Look for frozen entrees or dinners with:

About 300 to 400 calories per serving

No more than 3 grams of fat per 100 calories

Less than 800 milligrams of sodium

Less than 100 milligrams of cholesterol

▲ EXPANDED FOOD LIST ▲

Convenience Foods

FOOD	QUANTITY	EXCHANGES
Frozen Dinners:		
Dinners	11 oz.	2 starch/bread
		1 vegetable
		2 to 3 med. fat meat
		1 fat

FOOD	QUANTITY	EXCHANGES
Dinners	16 oz.	3 starch/bread 1 vegetable 3 med. fat meat 3 fat
Oriental Dinners	1½ cup	1 starch/bread 1 vegetable 2 lean meat
Light Dinners: Classic Lite	11 oz.	1½ starch/bread 1 vegetable 2 lean meat
Gourmet Light & Healthy	11 oz.	1 to 2 starch/bread 1 vegetable 2 lean meat
Healthy Choice	11 oz.	2 starch/bread 1 vegetable 2 lean meat
Le Menu, Light Style	10 oz.	1 to 2 starch/bread 1 vegetable 2 lean meat
Lean Cuisine	10 oz.	1 to 2 starch/bread 1 vegetable 2 to 3 lean meat
Entrees: Bean and Cheese Burrito	5 oz.	3 starch/bread 1 med. fat meat 1 fat
Chili with Beans	10.5 oz.	2 starch/bread 2 med. fat meat 1 fat
Cookin' Bags	4 oz.	½ starch/bread 1 med. fat meat
Family Entrees	8 oz.	2 starch/bread 1 to 2 med. fat meat
French Bread Pizza	6.25 oz.	3 starch/bread 2 med. fat meat
Hamburger Helper	1 cup	2 starch/bread 2 med. fat meat 1 fat

FOOD	QUANTITY	EXCHANGES
Lite Entrees	9 oz.	2 starch/bread 1 vegetable 2 lean meat
Lunch Bucket	8½ oz.	1 to 2 starch/bread 1 med. fat meat
Macaroni and Cheese	¾ cup	2 starch/bread 1 med. fat meat 1 fat
Meat Pies	7 oz.	2 starch/bread 1 vegetable 1 to 2 med. fat meat 4 to 5 fat
Microcup Entrees	7.5 oz.	1 to 2 starch/bread 1 to 2 med. fat meat 1 fat
Oriental Entrees	13 oz.	3 to 4 starch/bread 1 lean meat
Oriental Light Entrees	11.25 oz.	2 starch/bread 1 vegetable 1 lean meat
Pasta Classics	12 oz.	3 starch/bread 1 vegetable 2 lean meat
Pizzas, frozen	¼ of 23 oz.	2 starch/bread 2 med. fat meat 1 to 2 fat
Spaghetti Dinner	1 cup	2 to 3 starch/bread 1 med. fat meat 1 fat
Tuna Noodle Casserole	10 oz.	2 starch/bread 2 med. fat meat
Tuna Helper	1 cup	2 starch/bread 1½ lean meat 1 fat
Accompaniments:		
Noodles and Sauce	½ cup	1½ starch/bread 1 fat
Noodles Romanoff	½ cup	1 starch/bread 1 med. fat meat 1 fat

FOOD	QUANTITY	EXCHANGES
Potatoes, Au Gratin	½ cup	1½ starch/bread 1 fat
Potatoes, Scalloped	½ cup	1 starch/bread 1 fat
Potato Salad	½ cup	1 starch/bread 2 fat
Rice, Fried with Chicken and Pork	1 cup	3 starch/bread 1 fat
Rice, microwave dishes	½ cup	2 starch/bread
Stuffing Mix, microwave	½ cup	1½ starch/bread 1 fat
Suddenly Salads	½ cup	1½ starch/bread 1 to 2 fat
Tater Tots, all varieties	3 oz.	1 starch/bread 1½ fat
Twice Baked Potatoes	5 oz.	2 starch/bread 2 fat
Breads:		
Breadstix, average	6	1 starch/bread
Croissants	1	1½ starch/bread 3 fat
Croissants, petite	1	1 starch/bread 1½ fat
Dinner Rolls	1	1 starch/bread ½ fat
Light Muffins	1	1 starch/bread
Muffins	1	1 to 1 ½ starch/bread 1 fat
Quick Bread Mixes	⅟₁₆ loaf	1 starch/bread 1 fat
Soups:		
Chunky Soups (10 ¾ oz.)	1 can	1 starch/bread 1 vegetable 1 med. fat meat
Cup-A-Soup (broth-type)	6 oz.	½ starch/bread
(country-style)	6 oz.	1 starch/bread
Cup O Noodles	1 container	2 starch/bread 3 fat

FOOD	QUANTITY	EXCHANGES
Microcup Hearty	7.5 oz.	1 starch/bread 1 lean meat
Ramen Noodle	1 container	2½ starch/bread 2 fat
Ramen Noodle, low-fat	1 container	3 starch/bread
Desserts:		
Almost Home Cookies, all varieties	2 (1 oz.)	1 starch/bread 1 fat
American Collection Cookies, all varieties	1	1 starch/bread 1 fat
Fat-Free Cakes	1 oz. slice	1 starch/bread
Frozen Dairy Dessert	4 oz.	1½ starch/bread
Frookies Cookies, all varieties	2	1 starch/bread 1 fat
Gingersnaps	3	1 starch/bread ½ fat
Kitchen Hearth Cookies	3	1 starch/bread 1½ fat
Lovin' Lites Cake, all varieties	½ cake	2 starch/bread
Supermoist Cake, all varieties	½ cake	2 starch/bread 2 fat
Breakfast Items:		
Egg Beaters	½ cup	1 lean meat
French Toast, frozen	2 slices	2 starch/bread ½ med. fat meat
Pancakes, mix	3, 4" cakes	2 starch/bread 1 fat
Pancakes, microwave	2 cakes	2 starch/bread
Waffles, frozen	1	1 starch/bread ½–1 fat
Beverages:		
Hot Cocoa Mixes (sugar free)	1 package	1 starch/bread **or** 1 skim milk

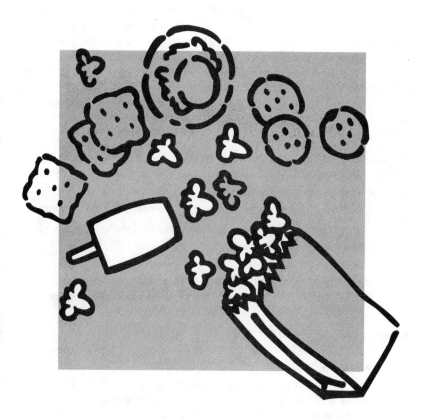

EXCHANGES FOR
SMART SNACKING

Although snacking often has a "bad name," snacks can add important nutrients and enjoyment to a meal plan. However, snacks can also contribute a significant amount of fat, salt, and calories to the diets of many people. Sale of salty snacks is a $6.1 billion industry. The average American household is reported to consume 28.6 pounds of salty snacks per year: 44 percent in potato chips, 24 percent in corn tortilla chips, 15 percent from salted nuts, 5 percent each from salted meat snacks, pretzels, and other salted snacks, and 2 percent in popcorn.

The following are hints for choosing snack foods:

▲ Choose your foods carefully. Avoid empty calorie snacks that are high in sugar, fat, salt, and calories, but low in nutrients.

▲ Buy or prepare snacks that are low in fat and salt. If high-fat and salt snacks are not in the house, they will not be consumed.

▲ When you have time to prepare your own snacks, modify your recipes. Cut down the amount of sugar and use skim milk, margarine, oils, egg whites, or egg substitutes.

▲ When preparing snacks, try seasoning with spices such as basil, dill, lemon juice, and garlic or onion powder instead of salt.

▲ If you are trying to control your weight, avoid nuts, seeds, dried fruits, and modified sweets that may be healthful but not necessarily helpful in reducing calories.

▲ Snack on foods that contain carbohydrates and fiber. They contribute nutrients, such as vitamins and minerals, along with fiber. Keep fruits and vegetables on hand in the refrigerator. They make excellent snacks.

▲ Beware of commercially manufactured snack bars, energy bars, and other snack foods. They are frequently similar to candy bars and often are scarcely more than fat, sugar, and salt with a little flavoring.

▲ Examine the ingredient list and nutrition label on purchased snack items. Try to find snacks that have 3 or fewer grams of fat per serving.

▲ Plan ahead to make sure you have appropriate and appealing snacks available.

▲ If your meal plan includes snacks, don't skip them. Use a snack that fits into your number of meal plan exchanges. Substitute snacks containing sugar for starch/bread or fruit exchanges. Watch the portion size.

▲

Healthy Snack Choice Ideas

Bread or toast (whole grain), bagels, English muffins, breadsticks
Cereal snack mix (prepare with garlic powder, Worcestershire sauce, and margarine)
Cookies (homemade with whole grains, oils, and minimal sugar)
Crackers
No-fat commercial choices: Finn Crisps, flatbread, hardtack, Matzo, Wasa Brod, Akmak
Low-fat commercial choices: bread sticks, melba toast, RyKrisps, zwieback, graham crackers, oyster crackers, saltines
Dried fruits: apricots, dates, prunes, raisins
Frozen yogurt
Frozen fruit or yogurt bars
Fruits and fruit juices (fresh, frozen, or canned in fruit juice)
Fruit and nut breads (prepared with whole grains, oils, and minimal sugar)
Fruit jerky, fruit roll-ups, and fruit bars
Fruited yogurts, artificially sweetened
Low-fat commercial snacks: animal crackers, gingersnaps, fig bars, graham crackers, molasses cookies
Popcorn (air-popped or microwave light, served plain, lightly salted, or sprinkled with Parmesan cheese)
Pretzels
Sandwiches
Trail mix (popcorn, raisins, peanuts, dates, and dried fruits such as apricots, peaches, pears, and pineapple)
Vegetables (raw, cooked, or served with low-fat dips)

For additional snack ideas and recipes see *The Joy of Snacks* by Nancy Cooper, R.D., C.D.E.

If you have diabetes, especially if you take injected insulin, you can eat snacks that can be helpful in the regulation of blood glucose levels. Without a snack, your blood glucose levels can easily drop too low, causing hypoglycemia. The need to snack depends on your insulin regime, age, activity level, and calorie needs. In general, children and active adults using injected insulin do well with a mid-morning, mid-afternoon, and bedtime snack. Some kids do even better with two afternoon snacks, depending on the times of their school lunch and dinner. Most persons who use insulin need an afternoon and evening snack to keep their blood glucose stable over these longer spans of time.

In addition to knowing when to snack, you also need to know what and how much to eat. Eating too much or an inappropriate snack can cause blood glucose levels to soar and can also contribute more calories than you need.

Sometimes what is healthy and best just isn't convenient! For such occasions, the following "legal junk foods" can help you make the best choice available. It's important to weigh convenience and neccessity against the ideal—there are times when you will go with convenience. This list can help with those occasions!

▲ EXPANDED FOOD LIST ▲

Snacks

FOOD	QUANTITY	EXCHANGES
Starch/Bread:		
Breads:		
Bread sticks, hard	6	1 starch/bread
4" long, 1/4" diameter		
Cocktail/Party rye bread	4 slices	1 starch/bread
Fat Free fruit muffins,	1	1 starch/bread
all varieties		1 fruit

FOOD	QUANTITY	EXCHANGES
Wholesome Choice muffins, all varieties	1	2 starch/bread
Popcorn cakes, regular	2 cakes	1 starch/bread
Mini size	8 cakes	1 starch/bread
Rice cakes, regular	2 cakes	1 starch/bread
Mini size	½ oz.	1 starch/bread
Chips and Snacks:		
Chex Mix	½ cup	1 starch/bread ½ fat
Corn chips, all varieties	34	1 starch/bread 2 fat
Cornnuts	¾ oz.	1 starch/bread 1 fat
DooDads	½ cup	1 starch/bread 1 fat
Granola bar, plain (not dipped or coated)	1	1 starch/bread 1 fat
Munch'Ems-cheddar	26 crackers	1 starch/bread 1 fat
Nutri-Grain cereal bars	1 bar	1 starch/bread 1 fruit 1 fat
Oriental mix, rice-based	1 oz.	1 starch/bread 2 fat
Popcorn, cheese-flavor	1 oz.	1 starch/bread 2 fat
Popcorn, hot air	5 cups	1 starch/bread
Popcorn, microwave, natural/butter	5 cups	1 starch/bread 2 fat
Popcorn, light	5 cups	1 starch/bread
Potato chips all varieties	1 oz.	1 starch/bread 2 fat
Potato chips, light	1 oz.	1 starch/bread 1 fat
Pretzels, rods	1	1 starch/bread
sticks, very thin	65	1 starch/bread
twists, 3-ring	4	1 starch/bread
Sesame sticks	1 oz.	1 starch/bread 2 fat

FOOD	QUANTITY	EXCHANGES
Snack Crisps (Estee), all varieties	1 bag	1 starch/bread
Snack cracker mixes	⅓ cup (1 oz.)	1 starch/bread 1 fat
Snacklin cheddar cracker	27 crackers	1 starch/bread 1 fat
Snackwells-cinnamon graham snacks	14 crackers	1 starch/bread
Sun chips	1 small bag	1 starch/bread 1½ fat
Taro chips	¾ oz.	1 starch/bread 1 fat
Tortilla chips, all varieties	15 to 18	1 starch/bread 1 fat
Trail mix (raisin, nuts, coconut, dried fruit)	¼ cup	1 starch/bread 1 fat
Trail mix (with chocolate chips)	¼ cup	1 starch/bread 2 fat
Trail mix, tropical	¼ cup	1 starch/bread 1 fat
Cookies:		
Mini Chips Ahoy	9	1 starch/bread 1 fat
Cookies, in general	1, 3" diameter, 1	1 starch/bread 1 fat
Fig Newtons or bars	2	1½ starch/bread
Frookie,		
Apple or Fig Fruitins	1	1 fruit
Cinnamon and Chocolate Animal Frackers	10 cookies	1 starch/bread 1 fat
Fat-Free Cookies	2	1 starch/bread
Frookwich	2 cookies	1 starch/bread 1 fat
Frookies	2 cookies	1 starch/bread 1 fat
Fat-Free Crackers	8	1 starch/bread
Cool Fruits	2 squeezers	1 fruit
Funky Mountains	12	1 starch/bread
Gingersnaps	3	1 starch/bread
Lorna Doone shortbread	6	1 starch/bread 1½ fat

FOOD	QUANTITY	EXCHANGES
Oatmeal raisin cookies	2	1 starch/bread 1 fat
Vanilla wafers	6	1 starch/bread
Crackers:		
Animal crackers	7	1 starch/bread
Cheese Nips	20	1 starch/bread 1 fat
Cheez 'n Crackers	1 package	½ starch/bread ½ med. fat meat 1 fat
Chex Mix, traditional	½ cup	1 starch/bread 1 fat
Chicken in a Biskit	14 (1 oz.)	1 starch/bread 2 fat
Dinosaur grahams, large	1	1 starch/bread
Garden Crisps, vegetable	11 crackers	1 starch/bread ½ fat
Goldfish, all varieties	45	1 starch/bread 1 fat
Harvest Crisps, 5-Grain & Oat	12 crackers	1 starch/bread 1 fat
Melba toast	5 slices	1 starch/bread
Melba rounds	8 rounds	1 starch/bread
Peanut Butter 'n Cheez	1 package	1 starch/bread ½ med. fat meat 2 fat
Ritz or Hi Ho crackers	6	1 starch/bread 1 fat
Ritz Bits	40	1 starch/bread 1 fat
Teddy Grahams	15	1 starch/bread ½ fat
Wheat or Vegetable Thins	14 crackers	1 starch/bread 1 fat
Wheatables	24 (1 oz.)	1 starch/bread 1 fat
Frozen Desserts:		
Baskin Robbins Truly Free Frozen Yogurt	½ cup	1 starch/bread

FOOD	QUANTITY	EXCHANGES
Frozen Yogurt	⅓ cup	1 starch/bread
Soft-Serve Sorbet	⅓ cup	1 starch/bread
Sugar Free Low, Lite 'n Luscious	½ cup	1 starch/bread
Light	½ cup	1 starch/bread 1 fat
Fat Free	⅓ cup	1 starch/bread
Ice Cream	1 regular scope	2 starch/bread 3 fat
Dairy Queen Cone	small	1½ starch/bread 1 fat
DQ sandwich	1	1½ starch/bread 1 fat
Eskimo Pie		
Regular	1	1 starch/bread 2 fat
Sugar Freedom	1	1 starch/bread 2 fat
Sugar Freedom Sandwiches	1	1½ starch/bread 1 fat
Fruit ices	½ cup	1 starch/bread
Fudgesicle, sugar-free	1	½ starch/bread
Gelatin Pops	1	½ starch/bread
Ice cream	~4 oz. cup	1 starch/bread 1 fat
Ice cream, soft-serve	½ cup	1 starch/bread 2 fat
Ice milk	½ cup	1 starch/bread 1 fat
Ice milk, soft-serve	½ cup	1 starch/bread 1 fat
Ice pops	1 bar	½ fruit
Kemps Lite Ice Milk Sandwich	1	1½ starch/bread ½ fat
Nestle Crunch Sugar Free, Reduced Fat Vanilla Lite Bar	1	1 starch/bread 2 fat
Pudding Pop	1	1 starch/bread
Simple Pleasures Toffee Crunch	½ cup	1½ starch/bread 2 fat
Yogurt, frozen, all varieties	⅓ cup	1 starch/bread

FOOD	QUANTITY	EXCHANGES
Yogurt, nonfat frozen, all varieties	½ cup	1 starch/bread
Yogurt, soft-serve	½ cup	1 starch/bread 1 fat
Yoplait		
Soft Frozen Yogurt Cup	1 (3 oz.)	1 starch/bread
Sugar-Free, Triple-Dipped Dairy Dessert	1 bar	1 starch/bread 1 fat
Soup:		
Cup-A-Soup		
Broth-type	6 oz.	½ starch/bread
Cream-type	6 oz.	½ starch/bread 1 fat
Country Style	6 oz.	1 starch/bread
Lite	6 oz.	½ starch/bread
Fruit:		
All Fruit spreads	1 tablespoon	1 fruit
Applesauce, unsweetened	½ cup	1 fruit
Dried fruit	¼ cup, (½ oz.)	1 fruit
Dried fruit pouch	1 pouch	1 fruit
Fruit bars	1	1 fruit
Fruit by the Foot	1 roll	1 fruit
Fruit Jerkey	1 strip	1 fruit
Fruit juice bars	1 (3 ox.)	1 fruit
Fruit Sorbet/Sherbet, all varieties	½ cup	2 fruit **or** 1 starch/bread
Fruit Roll-Ups	1 (½ oz.)	1 fruit
Fruit Wrinkles	1 pouch	1½ fruit
Fun Fruits	1 pouch	1½ fruit
Mama Tish's Sugar-Free Italian Ice	½ cup	1 fruit
Raisins	½ oz. box	1 fruit
Weight Watcher Fruit Snacks	1 package, (½ oz.)	1 fruit
Gushers	1 pouch	1 fruit
Juices:		
Apple cider	½ cup	1 fruit
Catawba juice	½ cup	1 fruit
Cranberry juice cocktail	⅓ cup	1 fruit

FOOD	QUANTITY	EXCHANGES
Fruit nectars, apricot, peach, pear	⅓ cup	1 fruit
Gatorade	1 cup	1 fruit
Low-calorie Hawaiian punch, cranberry juice cocktail, cranapple drink	1 cup	1 fruit
Sundance sparkling water with fruit juice	5 oz.	1 fruit
Tomato juice, vegetable juice cocktail	1 cup	1 fruit
Meats:		
Meat, Poultry, Fish:		
Beef jerky	2 **or** ½ oz.	1 lean meat
Buddig meats	1 oz.	1 lean meat
Cheese:		
Cheez Whiz	2 tablespoons	1 med. fat meat
Cottage cheese, low-fat/nonfat	¼ cup	1 lean meat
Diet cheeses: Light & Lively, Lite-Line, Weight Watchers	1 oz.	1 lean meat
Laughing Cow reduced calorie cheese spread	1 wedge (1 oz.)	1 lean meat
String cheese	1 oz.	1 med. fat meat
Velveeta slices/spread	1 oz.	1 high fat meat
Chunk chicken in water	1 oz.	1 lean meat
Chunk turkey in water	1 oz.	1 lean meat
Deli Select meats	1 oz.	1 lean meat
Nuts/Seeds	¼ cup, (1 oz.)	1 med. fat meat 2 fat
Peanut butter	1 tablespoon	1 high fat meat
Pickled herring	1 oz.	1 med. fat meat
Salmon-pink, canned	1 oz.	1 lean meat
Sardines, medium	2	1 lean meat
Tuna, canned in water	1 oz.	1 lean meat
Milk:		
Alba 66 or 77	1 envelope	1 skim milk
Diet Instant Breakfast sweetened with NutraSweet	1 envelope, mixed with 1 cup skim milk	1 starch/bread 1 skim milk

FOOD	QUANTITY	EXCHANGES
Chocolate low-fat milk with NutraSweet	1 cup	1 skim milk ½ fat
Sugar-Free hot cocoa mix	1 envelope (6 oz.)	½ skim milk **or** ½ starch/bread
D-zerta reduced calorie pudding	½ cup	1 skim milk **or** 1 starch/bread
Jello sugar-free pudding	½ cup	1 skim milk **or** 1 starch/bread
Yogurt sweetened with NutraSweet, or light yogurt, lowfat or nonfat	1 container	1 skim milk

Fat:

Light cream cheese	2 tablespoons	1 fat
Weight Watchers cream cheese	2 tablespoons	1 fat
3 Musketeers snack bar, sugar-free	1 bar	1 fat

Free:

Bouillon beef broth	1 cup	Free
Cup-A-Broth	6 oz.	Free
Comet ice cream cones	1	Free
Crystal Light frozen juice bars	1	Free
Cool Whip lite whipped topping	2 tablespoons	Free
Dietetic syrups	1 tablespoon	Free
Estee dietetic gummy bears	2	Free
Estee dietetic hard candy	1	Free
Lean cream dip, all varieties	1 tablespoon	Free
Sugar-Free drink mix	8 oz. = 4 cal.	Free
Sugar-Free jello	1 cup	Free
Sugar-Free popsicle	1	Free
Sugar-Free Quik	1 teaspoon	Free
Salsa, all varieties	2 tablespoons	Free
Sour Lean sour cream	1 tablespoon	Free
Vegetables, raw	1 cup	Free

P A R T

3

GUIDELINES FOR FOOD PURCHASING AND PREPARATION

• • • • • •

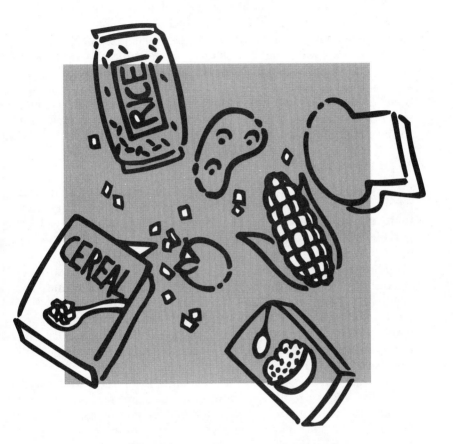

ADDING FIBER TO
YOUR MEAL PLAN

Fiber has been part of our diet since the beginning of time. Your grandmother may have called it "roughage" or "bulk." Although not new, its importance has been recognized only since the 1960s. In the 1980s fiber became a "cure-all" for all health problems. Today fiber is still an important part of the diet, but not a cure-all for all problems. Foods high in fiber have valuable health benefits. But equally as important, foods containing fiber also contain other nutrients—vitamins and minerals—that are important. At the same time, foods high in fiber are also low in fat.

What Is Fiber?

First, what is fiber? A type of carbohydrate, fiber is the structural part (or cell wall) of fruits, vegetables, grains, nuts, and legumes that can't be digested or broken down in the human digestive tract and absorbed into the bloodstream. Because of this, fiber does not contribute calories to the diet. There are two types of dietary fiber—insoluble and soluble—and each has specific benefits. Most fiber-containing foods contain both types of fiber, but often one type predominates and determines the characteristics of that food.

Insoluble fiber gives plants structure. It's called insoluble because it does not dissolve in water. It adds bulk to the diet and has a laxative effect on the digestive system. You usually feel fuller after eating foods containing insoluble fiber as well. Common sources are wheat and corn bran, whole grains, nuts, and some vegetables and fruits. Insoluble fibers are able to retain large amounts of water, thus increasing the volume of the stool and making it pass faster through the intestinal tract. Therefore, these fibers help prevent and treat constipation and diverticulosis, and many even help to prevent certain types of cancer, such as cancer of the colon and rectum.

Soluble fibers form a gel because they are soluble in water. They include fibers found in oats, legumes, barley, seeds, and some fruits and vegetables, particularly those with edible peels and seeds. Most soluble fibers are found within plant cells. The gummy texture of oat bran and the mushy center of a cooked kidney bean reflect the soluble fiber content and the ability of soluble fibers to soak up water. Soluble fibers can bind bile salts, cholesterol, and other sterols, thus reducing their absorption from the intestinal tract. These fibers have been found to lower cholesterol, especially when added to a low-fat diet. They may also offer some improvement in carbohydrate metabolism in people with diabetes.

It is a good idea to include foods in the diet with both soluble and insoluble fibers, because both are important for health. The following chart lists sources of fiber:

▲

Sources of Fiber

Richer in Insoluble Fiber:	Both Soluble and Insoluble Fiber:	Richer in Soluble Fiber:
wheat bran	oat bran	citrus fruits
whole wheat products	whole-grain oats	psyllium (Metamucil)
corn bran	barley	pectin
brown rice	navy beans	carrageenan
rice bran	soybeans	guar gum
bananas	kidney beans	
cauliflower	apples	
nuts	potatoes	
lentils	broccoli	
green beans	carrots	
green peas		

Why Eat Fiber?

Interest in fiber began in the 1960s when an English doctor, Denis Burkitt, reported on rural Africans whose diets were high in fiber. They had a much lower incidence of colon cancer, diverticulosis, hemorrhoids, gallstones, appendicitis, diabetes, and some forms of heart disease than Americans or Europeans.

Studies generally indicate a positive relationship between a high-fiber diet and decreased risk of disease, although it has been difficult to separate the effects of fiber from other dietary and lifestyle factors that also play a role in health. For example, people who eat more fiber tend to also eat less fat. It is the total dietary pattern; namely eating a diet high in grains, vegetables, and fruits—which is also a diet that's high in fiber—and low in fat, that has been linked to a reduced risk of disease and to good health.

Fiber is thought to be beneficial for certain health problems.

Gastrointestinal problems. Large amounts of insoluble fibers increase stool bulk and draw water into the large intestine. The result is a larger, softer stool that exerts less pressure on the colon walls and is eliminated more quickly. The most well-established benefit of a high-fiber diet is in the treatment and prevention of constipation. Constipation can contribute to hemorrhoids, varicose veins, and diverticular disease of the colon.

Cancer. If food contains carcinogens (cancer-causing agents), fiber speeds up transit time of stools through the digestive system, thus reducing exposure of the intestinal wall to those substances. Large amounts of insoluble fibers dilute the concentration of potential carcinogens that may be present in the stool, and the insoluble fibers also interfere with microbial activity that produces carcinogens. Both the National Cancer Institute and the American Cancer Society have recommended low-fat diets generous in dietary fiber to reduce the risk of colon, rectal, breast, and prostate cancer.

Obesity. Diets high in fiber can promote long-term weight loss and maintenance of that loss because foods containing fiber are typically low in fat and generally take longer to chew, thus slowing food intake. They also slow the emptying of foods from the stomach, contributing to the feeling of fullness, and since fiber is nondigestible it contributes practically no calories.

Coronary heart disease. Diets rich in soluble fibers have been shown to lower total blood cholesterol levels and low-density lipoprotein (LDL) cholesterol in people with both high and normal blood cholesterol levels. Soluble fibers appear to reduce blood cholesterol in two ways. First, they prevent the reabsorption of bile acids from the small intestine. To replace the lost bile acids, cholesterol is drawn from the body, thereby reducing its cholesterol supply. Second, the fermentation of soluble fibers in the intestine produces short-chain fatty acids that block the manufacture of cholesterol by the body. They also raise levels of high-density lipoproteins (HDL or "good" cholesterol), which are protective against heart disease.

Hypertension. Some evidence also suggests that dietary fiber may lower blood pressure.

Diabetes. Some studies suggest soluble fibers may help control the rise in blood glucose levels following a meal and reduce insulin requirements. Soluble fibers may slow emptying of foods from the stomach, slowing the absorption of glucose in the process. Although the studies are inconclusive, people with diabetes should include fiber in their diets for the same health reasons that all Americans should.

How Much Fiber Should You Consume?

Estimates currently indicate that the average dietary fiber intake is between 10 to 30 grams a day, with men averaging 19 grams a day and women 13 grams. The National Cancer Institute advises an increase to 20 to 35 grams a day. Consumption of both types of fiber should be increased by eating more foods from all the vegetable, grain, and fruit sources. The Diet and Health report of the National Academy of Sciences has gone one step further by specifying recommended amounts of foods high in fiber. It advises a daily intake of five or more servings of fruits and vegetables and six or more servings of whole grain breads and cereals and legumes. Fiber supplements are not recommended as a way to meet dietary guidelines.

It is important not to go overboard with an immediate leap from a low-fiber intake to recommended levels. Increasing fiber too rapidly can cause flatulence (gas), cramping, diarrhea, or bloating. Undesirable side effects may be avoided through the gradual addition of fiber to the diet along with adequate amounts of liquids.

Although concerns that fiber may interfere with the absorption of some minerals have been expressed, studies show people who consume well-balanced and varied diets high in fiber are unlikely to experience mineral deficiencies.

An added benefit of eating a high fiber diet is that, although fiber is classified as a carbohydrate and therefore is included on food labels as total carbohydrate, it is nondigestible and contributes virtually no calories. The grams of carbohydrate from fiber are not included in the caloric calculation.

The following tips can help you add more of both types of fiber to your diet.

Guidelines

▲ **Increase your fiber intake slowly.** Digestive discomfort from intestinal gas may occur when fiber intake is increased. Generally, this is only a temporary problem and will subside as the body adjusts to a higher fiber diet. This problem can be minimized by increasing fiber intake gradually. Start with small servings and increase portions gradually.

▲ **Eat a variety of fiber-rich foods in reasonable amounts.** Increase your intake of whole grain breads and cereals. Cereals can be an excellent source of fiber and make good choices for breakfast. Choose whole grain cereals, such as bran flakes and other high-fiber varieties, instead of low-fiber, high-fat breakfast items. Other good choices are oatmeal, cornmeal, corn tortillas, pumpernickel, rice cakes, popcorn, wheat germ, and bulgur.

Eat five or more servings daily of fruits and vegetables. Frozen, canned, or dried fruits and vegetables can be kept on hand and become staples in your diet. Excellent choices are citrus fruits, strawberries, and kiwi; deep yellow and dark green vegetables like carrots, greens, cantaloupe, tomatoes, and peppers; and cabbage-family vegetables including broccoli, cauliflower, and bok choy.

▲ **Try to drink six to eight glasses of water a day.** Fiber attracts water, so it's important to drink enough liquids when you add fiber to your diet.

▲ **Switch from white bread to whole grain varieties, such as whole wheat and rye.** Choose products made from stone ground flour, 100% whole wheat, or other whole grain flours. They should be the first ingredient on the label. "Brown-colored" breads contain little or no whole grain, just molasses for coloring. If the label says "wheat flour" remember almost all flours are made from wheat, and this phrase usually refers to bleached, white flour. You get the most nutrients and the best flavor from stone-ground, whole-wheat flour. Second best is ordinary whole-wheat flour. You can also buy whole-wheat pastry flour.

▲ **Select whole fresh fruit and vegetables instead of juices— they contain much more fiber.** Eat the skin of cleaned fruit (such as apples), membranes (such as oranges), or seeds (such as strawberries). Include more raw and slightly cooked vegetables such as corn, peas, beans, legumes, and potatoes with the skin. The stems and leaves of salad greens and broccoli are also fibrous. Don't throw away these good fiber sources. Add dry beans and peas to soups, stews, and casseroles. Use these legumes as main dishes, along with whole wheat pasta.

▲ **Go for carbohydrates packaged in their natural fibrous coatings.** Examples are brown rice instead of white rice; whole-grain flours instead of white flour; peelings on fruits and vegetables; whole fruits instead of juice; baked potatoes with skin instead of mashed potatoes.

▲ **Choose high-fiber, low-fat snacks.** Snack on vegetables, fruit, air-popped popcorn, and cereals, rather than cakes, cookies, and chocolate.

▲ **Watch calories.** If you add extra calories by adding high-fiber foods to your daily eating instead of substituting them for other food choices, you will probably gain weight. To save calories, trim your intake of high-fat, high-calorie foods such as cream, gravies, sauces, salad dressings, and other fats and oils. Eat breads and vegetables without margarine or butter; use noncaloric products (such as Pam) for "greasing" pans; use nonstick pans. Choose lean meats and do not exceed the recommended amount (usually four to six ounces a day).

▲ **Unless prescribed by your doctor, your fiber source should be food, not fiber supplements.** Fiber supplements usually do not contain large amounts of dietary fiber, nor do they have all the nutrients that accompany fiber in foods. Metamucil is an example of a fiber supplement. It is made from the husks of a seed grain called psyllium that is especially rich in soluble fiber. Although safe to use, it is more important to eat a diet that includes a wide variety of high-fiber foods.

How Do You Plan Fiber-Containing Meals?

Now you know the basics of high-fiber eating, but how do you plan meals? *Exchange Lists for Meal Planning* can help you. A symbol for fiber has been placed next to foods that contain three grams or more of dietary fiber per serving. Servings from the fruit, vegetable, and the whole-grain breads and crackers lists have two grams of dietary fiber. To help you choose foods high in fiber the following is a general guide giving you average values for foods on the exchange list.

▲ List 1. Starch/Bread

Cereals:
One serving (½–¾ cup) of fiber-containing cereals—either dry or cooked—averages 2 to 3 grams of fiber.
> *Examples: Cheerios, Nutri-Grains, Total, Wheaties, Grape-Nuts, Grape-Nuts Flakes, Oatmeal*

One serving (½–¾ cup) of fiber-containing cereals—either dry or cooked—averages 4 to 5 grams of fiber.
> *Examples: Bran Flakes, Fiberwise, Shredded Wheat, Oat Bran, Corn Bran, Wheatena*

One serving (⅓–½ cup) of bran cereals averages 8 to 12 grams of fiber.
> *Examples: Fiber One, All-Bran, All-Bran with Extra Fiber, 100% Bran, Bran Buds*

Breads and Crackers:
One serving (1 slice or 1 oz.) of whole-grain or whole-wheat breads and crackers averages 2 grams of fiber.

Grains:
One serving (½ cup) of grains such as kasha, couscous, bulgur, brown rice, or wild rice averages 2 grams of fiber.

Starchy Vegetables:
One serving (½ cup) of starchy vegetables such as corn, lima beans, green peas, or potatoes averages 3 grams of fiber.

Dried Beans, Peas, Lentils:
One serving (⅓ cup) of legumes such as dried, cooked peas, beans, or lentils averages 4 to 5 grams of fiber.

▲ List 2. Meat and Meat Substitutes

Meat and meat products do not contain any significant amount of fiber.
Nuts and Seeds:
One serving (½ oz. nuts or seeds) averages 2 grams of fiber.

▲ List 3. Vegetables

One serving (½–¾ cup) cooked, from canned or frozen, averages
2 grams of fiber.
One serving (1–2 cups) raw averages 3 grams of fiber.

▲ List 4. Fruits

A one-half cup serving of fresh, frozen, or canned fruit or one medium fruit
averages 2 grams of fiber.

▲ List 5. Milk

Milk products do not contain fiber.

▲ List 6. Fats

Fat products do not contain fiber.

SAMPLE MENU

▲ High Fiber, High Carbohydrate ▲

1,500 Calories

	Meal Plan (Exchanges)	Menu (Foods)	Fiber (Grams)
Breakfast:	2 starch/bread	⅔ cup All Bran	16
	1 fruit	1 medium orange	2
	½ skim milk	½ cup skim milk	0
Snack:	1 fruit	1 apple	2
Lunch:	2 starch/bread	2 slices whole-wheat bread	4
	1 meat	1 oz. sliced turkey	0
	1 vegetable	2 cups lettuce with reduced-calorie dressing	2
	1 fruit	15 grapes	2
	1 skim milk	1 cup skim milk	0
	1 fat	1 tsp. margarine	0
Snack:	1 starch/bread	4 squares RyKrisp	2
Dinner:	1 starch/bread	⅓ cup brown rice	2
	1 starch/bread	1 whole-wheat roll	2
	3 meat	3 oz. broiled fish	0
	1 vegetable	1 cup broccoli	2
	1 vegetable	2 cups spinach with reduced-calorie dressing	2
	1 fruit	⅓ cup pineapple chunks	2
	1 fat	1 tsp. margarine	0
Evening Snack:	1 starch/bread	3 cups popcorn, no butter	2
Totals:	1,500 calories	220 gms carbohydrate (61%)	
		75 gms protein (21%)	
		30 gms fat (18%)	
		42 gms of **FIBER**	

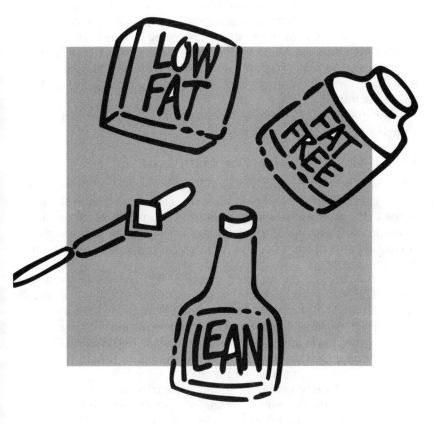

GOING LEAN—
CUTTING BACK ON FAT

More and more Americans are concerned about the amount of fat they are eating. The reason—coronary heart disease is the leading cause of death in the United States. Furthermore, one out of every four adults is overweight and is trying to lose weight. Diets high in fat influence blood cholesterol levels, are usually high in calories, and increase risk for some cancers. Dietary fat contributes more than twice as many calories as equal amounts (by weight) of either protein or carbohydrates.

The question today is how to cut back on fats in the diet and still have tasty foods that we can enjoy.

What Are The Different Types of Fat?

First, what is fat and what are the different types of fat? Dietary fats come from both plant and animal foods. They are an essential part of the diet and a major source of energy (calories). All types of fat have the same number of calories (9 calories per gram). Although fat is vital in order for the body to function properly, most Americans consume far more fat than they really need.

Fatty acids are the building blocks of fat, and there are three kinds of fatty acids—saturated, monounsaturated, and polyunsaturated. All foods that contain fat are made of mixtures of these fatty acids. Triglycerides—combinations of three of these fatty acids—are the way fat is found in foods. A food is classified as contributing saturated or unsaturated fat to the diet based on the type of fatty acids it contains in the largest amount.

Saturated fatty acids are found primarily in foods of animal origin, such as meat, dairy fat from food products such as cheeses and butter, and lard, and in foods from plant sources, coconut oil, palm oil, and palm kernel oil. They are usually solid at room temperature. A diet high in fat, especially saturated fats, can increase blood cholesterol levels, a risk factor for coronary heart disease.

Monounsaturated fatty acids are found in both animal and plant foods. Olive, peanut, and canola oils, avocados, and most nuts are high in monounsaturated fat and low in saturated fatty acids. Although poultry and beef also contain monounsaturated fats, they are primarily sources of saturated fats. When substituted for saturated fats, monounsaturated fats may help to lower blood cholesterol levels.

Polyunsaturated fatty acids are found mainly in oils from plants, such as safflower, sunflower, corn, soybean, and cottonseed oils. They also lower blood cholesterol levels. Cold-water fish, such as mackerel, perch, cod, salmon, tuna, and sole, and some fish oils contain special kinds of polyunsaturated fatty acids called *omega-3 fatty acids.* In countries where fish intake is high and saturated fat intake is low, the coronary heart disease rate is low. Because of this, it's recommended that we eat fish two or more times a week.

Hydrogenation is a process that changes fatty acids from liquid to more solid forms at room temperature. This makes it possible to use the oil in processed foods like margarines and baked products to extend their shelf life. Hydrogenation, however, also makes an oil more saturated.

Cholesterol is a fat-like, waxy substance. The body needs cholesterol to make hormones and to support and protect cells. Cholesterol is made by the body and in the diet comes from animal foods, such as meat, poultry, egg yolks, and dairy products. The effect of cholesterol in the diet on cholesterol in the blood varies from person to person.

The amount of saturated fats and total fat in the diet has more of an effect on blood cholesterol levels than cholesterol in food. Even though foods do not contain cholesterol they may be high in total and saturated fat, which is more of a concern.

Lipoproteins transport fats and cholesterol throughout the bloodstream to the cells where they can be used or stored. There are several kinds of lipoproteins, but two are especially important in determining risk for coronary heart disease: low-density lipoprotein (LDL) and high-density lipoprotein (HDL).

LDL-cholesterol carries most of the cholesterol throughout the body. When there is too much LDL-cholesterol in the bloodstream, it combines with other substances to form a plaque and narrows the blood vessels. When this happens, less blood reaches the heart and a coronary heart attack can happen. A high level of LDL-cholesterol increases the risk of coronary heart disease.

HDL-cholesterol carries cholesterol away from the arteries and to the liver where the liver can dispose of it. Therefore, a high level of HDL-cholesterol, also known as "good" cholesterol, protects against heart disease and a low HDL-cholesterol level increases coronary heart disease risk.

Triglycerides are the way that fat is found in foods—combinations of three fatty acids, the way that fat travels through the bloodstream, and the way that fat is stored in fat cells for future use. Very-low-density lipoproteins (VLDL) carry triglycerides through the bloodstream.

Why Cut Back on Fats?

High intakes of total dietary fat are associated with increased risk for obesity, some types of cancer, gallbladder disease, and coronary heart disease. Several factors increase the chances of developing coronary heart disease. Three of the main factors that increase risk are cigarette smoking, high blood pressure, and high blood cholesterol. What you eat, particularly the type and amount of fat in the diet, influences blood cholesterol levels. Saturated fats in foods are the major dietary contributors to total blood cholesterol levels.

Most heart attacks occur in people with blood cholesterol levels between 200 and 240 mg/dl. Approximately half of all adults have total cholesterol levels above 200 mg/dl. For each 1% reduction in high levels of blood cholesterol, there is a 2% decrease in the risk of coronary heart disease.

How Much Fat Should You Eat?

At present, Americans consume about 37% to 40% of their total calories from fat and 14% from saturated fat. They also consume 350 to 450 mg of cholesterol each day. Recommendations stress that fat intake be decreased to 30% or less of total calories, saturated fat intake below 10% of calories, and cholesterol below 300 mg daily.

But what does 30% of total daily calories mean? For example, if you're eating 1,500 calories per day; multiply 1,500 by 30% to determine the maximum number of calories that should come from fat in one day (1,500 x .30 = 450 calories from fat). Because 1 gram of fat provides 9 calories, divide the calories from fat by 9 to see how many grams of fat you should have per day (450 divided by 9 = 50 grams fat/day).

Another way to determine how many grams of fat is 30% of the calories is the following: drop the 0 from the number of calories and divide the result by 3. For example, drop the 0 from 1,500 calories and divide the result—150—by 3. Fifty grams is the amount of fat you should try to limit your intake to per day.

▲

If Your Total Calories Are...	Your Total Grams of Fat Should Be...
1,200	40
1,500	50
1,800	60
2,500	83
3,000	100
3,500	117

Now that you know how to figure fat, you can put food labels to good use. Labels tell you how much fat is in each serving. This can help you keep track of your daily intake.

Guidelines

The following tips can help you decrease total fat, saturated fats, and cholesterol in your diet.

▲ **Limit meat exchanges**. Most adults should limit meat exchanges to six per day. Some women may need only four to five, persons on meal plans of more than 2,000 calories may be able to have eight.

▲ **Use lean meat exchanges whenever possible.** Today, many lower fat and reduced fat meat choices are available. Look for luncheon meats that have 3 or fewer grams of fat per ounce. See Chapter 4 for a listing of lean meat choices.

▲ **Avoid high-fat meat exchanges**. Regular luncheon and other processed meats, frankfurters, wieners, sausage, and bacon or prime cuts of meat are higher fat meat choices. Limit these to three or fewer times per week.

▲ **Add no extra fat in the preparation of foods and cook away as much fat as possible by baking, broiling, or roasting.** If pan frying meat, drain the fat as it cooks out; if meat remains in the fat while cooking, the fat is reabsorbed by the meat. Chill gravies, soups, or stews until the fat hardens, remove the fat layer, then reheat and serve.

▲ **Drink skim or 1% milk.**

▲ **Choose low-fat or nonfat dairy products.** Plain nonfat yogurt and skim milk cheeses are examples. Look for cheeses that have five or fewer grams of fat per ounce.

▲ **Use margarine instead of butter, but be careful of amounts.** Look for margarines that list a liquid oil such as corn, saf- flower, or soybean oil as the first ingredient. A soft or tub mar- garine is not as hydrogenated or saturated as a solid or stick margarine and is a good choice. The calories in magarine and butter are the same, but because butter contains more satu- rated fatty acids than margarine, margarine is recommended.

▲ **Substitute vegetable oils for hydrogenated solid shortenings whenever possible in baking and cooking and in salad dressings.** In most recipes, ¾ cup liquid vegetable oil may be substituted for 1 cup of solid shortening; ⅓ cup for ½ cup.

▲ **Choose reduced- or lower-calorie salad dressings.** If you pre- fer regular dressings, be very careful of the amount. One tablespoon of a reduced- or lower-calorie salad dressing may have less than 20 calories and be considered a "free" food, two to three tablespoons will be one fat exchange.

▲ **Substitute nonfat dry milk or condensed skim milk for cream or nondairy creamers if you use a coffee whitener.** They contain only 10 calories per teaspoon and are considered "free" foods. When using nonfat dry milk in hot beverages, allow the beverage to cool for a few minutes so the powder will dissolve without a curdled appearance.

Nondairy creamers contain about 20 calories for a ½ ounce of liquid, or 1½ teaspoons powdered portion. One portion may be considered "free" or equivalent to ½ fat exchange. However, these products are usually made from palm or coconut oils or other hydrogenated vegetable oils, which are saturated and therefore not recommended for use. If you use a whitener only once or twice a day, the amount of fat consumed will not be significant, but if you drink a significant amount of coffee each day and whiten it with a nondairy creamer, this may be a con- siderable amount of saturated fat.

▲ **Try some of the many "light" sour creams, mayonnaise, and salad dressings on the market.** They are made by using one of many fat substitutes. Carbohydrates or proteins are modified to have properties similar to fat and are used to replace fats in food products, replacing the nine calories of fat per gram with one to four calories from the carbohydrate or protein. Light and reduced- or low-calorie foods contain these substitutes. On the ingredient label, modified food starches, dextrins, cellulose gum or gel, microparticulated protein or texturized protein are examples of fat substitutes. See Chapter 26 for more information on fat substitutes.

▲ **Plain nonfat yogurt makes an excellent substitute for sour cream or mayonnaise in many recipes.** It is lower in calories and fat. Two tablespoons of plain yogurt have about 10 to 16 calories; two tablespoons of sour cream, 50 calories; and two tablespoons of mayonnaise, 200 calories.

If a recipe calls for cream, sweet or sour, or mayonnaise, substitute an equal amount of yogurt. To prevent yogurt from separating in cooking, mix one tablespoon of cornstarch with one tablespoon of yogurt. Stir this mixture into one cup of yogurt and heat over medium heat until thickened.

Recipe Modifications for Lowering Fat and Increasing Fiber

Now you know the basics of reducing fat in the diet, but how do you prepare foods at home to reduce total fat, saturated fat, and cholesterol? You can modify your recipes a number of ways to accomplish this, and you will reduce total calories, sodium, and/or added sugars at the same time. The two basic ways to modify a recipe are to change a cooking technique or an ingredient. An example of changing a cooking technique would be to saute vegetables in broth instead of in oil or butter, thus reducing total fat as well as the type of fat. You can modify ingredients by reducing them, eliminating them completely, or by substituting a more acceptable ingredient.

To reduce an ingredient, analyze the function of the ingredient in a recipe. Is it a necessary part of the final product, such as sugar in a cake? If so, you may not be able to reduce the amount used.

Products that can be eliminated are those added for appearance or because of habit and tradition. These products may be high in sodium or sugar.

Many substitutions can be made in recipes to lower the fat and cholesterol content. While taste and texture may change, the results are often just as pleasing. Remember—"The proof of the pudding is in the eating."

Possible substitutions to consider are:

▲ **Evaporated skim milk for cream.** However, in order to whip evaporated skim milk it must be partially frozen. Because of its thick consistency, evaporated skim milk also works well in cream sauces.

▲ **Skim milk for whole milk.**

▲ **Use two egg whites whipped in place of one egg or use egg substitutes for whole eggs.** However, some egg substitutes may have objectionable flavors. Flavor extracts may help disguise them.

▲ **Margarine for butter.** However, soft or tub margarines will not cream. Diet margarines contain more water and less fat and cannot be substituted ounce-per-ounce for butter.

▲ **Oils for hydrogenated fats (shortening).** However, crusts may not have the same flakiness, and dough may stick to rolling pins. Oils will not cream. One cup of shortening can be replaced by ¾ cup of oil; ½ cup of shortening by ⅓ cup oil. In some recipes it is the liquid that is important. In this case, you may be able to use ½ cup oil and ¼ cup of a liquid such as water, juice, or wine, in place of 1 cup of shortening.

▲ **Cocoa for chocolate.** You may also need to add some oil to the cocoa. Cocoa will not solidify to form a coating.

▲ **Whole grains for refined products.**

▲ **Reduce the fat in recipes by one-third to one-half.** In your favorite cake or soft-drop cookies recipe use no more than two tablespoons of fat per cup of flour; in muffin, quick bread, or biscuit recipes use no more than one to two tablespoons of fat per cup of flour; and in pie crust recipes use ½ cup margarine for two cups of flour.

▲ **Reduce amount of added sugars in recipes.** Sugar and other
sweeteners add flavor, color, tenderness, and crispness in
baked products. In many recipes you can reduce the amount
of sugar called for by at least ⅓ to ½ without affecting the quality of the product.

A helpful guideline: use no more than ¼ cup of added sweetener (sugar, honey, molasses, etc.) per one cup of flour.
Adding extra vanilla will enhance the sweetness of a recipe.
Vanilla, cinnamon, and nutmeg all give the illusion of sweetness without adding calories.

Persons with diabetes will generally enjoy their food products
the most when they use regular foods and learn to substitute for
them correctly in their meal plan. Sugar substitutes often do not
work well, especially in baked products. This is still true even if the
sugar substitute is heat-stable. Remember, just because a dessert
does not contain sugar does not mean it is a "free food." The calories
in the food product come from other ingredients—flour, eggs, shortening, and so on—that also raise blood glucose levels and require
insulin to be metabolized.

▲

Recipe Modifications and Substitutions for Lowering Fat, Added Sugars, and Salt and for Adding Fiber

Use this substitution information to modify your favorite recipes. They will be healthier but still look and taste as good as the original.

Ingredient	Recipe Modifications/Substitutions
Bacon, 2 strips	1 oz. lean Canadian bacon or 1 oz. lean ham
Bouillon cubes or granules	Low-sodium bouillon
Butter	Margarine; to cut total fat, reduce portions
Cheese, regular	Reduced-fat or skim milk cheese
Chocolate, baking, 1 oz. or 1 sq.	3 Tbsp. cocoa; if fat is needed to replace fat in chocolate, add 1 Tbsp. or less vegetable oil
Cream cheese	Light cream cheese **or** blend 4 Tbsp. margarine with 1 cut low-fat cottage cheese, salt to taste; small amount of skim milk is needed in blending.
Cream, heavy, 1 cup	1 cup evaporated skim milk **or** 1 cup Poly Perx **or** ⅔ cup skim milk and ⅓ cup oil
Cream, light	Equal portions of skim or 1% milk and evaporated skim milk
Egg, 1 whole	¼ cup egg substitute **or** 1 egg white + 1 tsp. vegetable oil **or** 2 egg whites whipped.
Evaporated milk	Evaporated skim milk
Fat in baked recipes	Use no more than 1–2 Tbsp. of added oil or fat per cup of flour. Increase low-fat moist or liquid ingredients, such as buttermilk, to add moistness; **or** replace ½ to ⅓ the oil in a recipe with: applesauce; babyfood fruits; or a mixture of 1 cup dried figs or dates pureed with ¾ cup water and 1 tsp. vanilla.
Flour, all-purpose, 1 cup	1 cup whole wheat flour minus amount of oil called for in recipe by 1 Tbsp. and increase liquid by 1–2 Tbsp.; **or** ½ cup white + ½ cup whole wheat flour; **or** ¾ cup white + ¼ cup wheat germ and/or bran.

Ingredient	Recipe Modifications/Substitutions
Frosting	Sprinkle powdered sugar
Fruit, syrup-packed, canned	Fruit, juice-packed, canned
Garlic, onion, and celery salt	Garlic, onion, and celery powder
Gelatin, regular	Sugar-free gelatin mix **or** fruit juice mixed with unflavored gelatin
Mayonnaise	Plain yogurt, add 1 Tbsp. mayo to each cup yogurt **or** use reduced-calorie mayonnaise
Milk, whole	Skim or 1% milk
Rice, white	Brown rice
Oil	Use a vegetable oil spray to keep foods from sticking
Salad dressing	Low- or reduced-calorie salad dressing
Salt in recipes	Reduce amount or eliminate, use spices and herbs
Shortening or lard, 1 cup	¾ cup vegetable oil **or** ½ cup vegetable oil, ¼ cup other liquid
Shortening, ½ cup	⅓ cup vegetable oil
Soup, condensed	Homemade skim milk white sauce (1 cup skim milk + 2 Tbsp. flour + 2 Tbsp. margarine)
Cream of celery, 1 can	1 cup sauce + ¼ cup chopped celery
Cream of chicken, 1 can	1 cup sauce + chicken bouillon powder
Cream of mushroom, 1 can	1 cup sauce + 1 small can drained mushrooms
Sour cream, 1 cup	1 cup nonfat plain yogurt **or** 1 cup low-fat cottage cheese with 2 Tbsp. lemon juice and 1 Tbsp. skim milk **or** "light" sour cream
Sugar in baked recipes	Reduce amount by up to ½ to ⅓ of the original amount; use no more than ¼ cup added sweetener (sugar, honey, molasses, etc.) per cup of flour.
Tuna or salmon, oil-packed	Water-packed tuna or salmon
Vegetables, canned with added salt	Fresh **or** frozen vegetables **or** low-salt canned or rinse canned vegetables

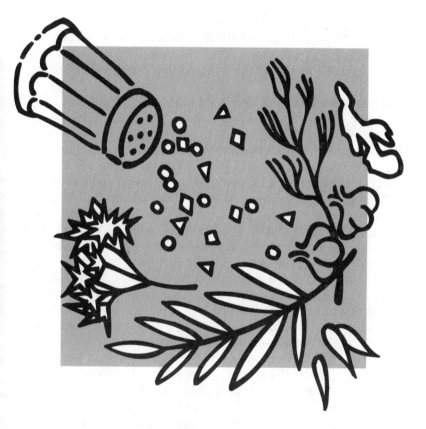

SPRINKLE LESS
SALT— CHOOSE NEW
SPICES

All Americans are encouraged to cut back on their sodium (salt) intake. Obesity, inherited tendency (genetics), and high salt intake increase the risk of developing high blood pressure (hypertension). High blood pressure is a serious health problem affecting about one of every four people. It is called "the silent killer" because it rarely produces warning signals, yet it can lead to serious problems.

Blood pressure is the force pushing blood through the body's circulatory system. High blood pressure, or hypertension, occurs when blood pushes against the walls of the arteries with extreme force. Because this puts extra strain on the heart, it's an important risk factor in coronary heart and blood vessel disease. Two other important factors are high blood cholesterol levels and smoking.

Blood pressure is measured using a device called a sphygmomanometer. That's the technical name for the inflatable cuff, bulb, and dial or column of mercury so familiar to many of us. The person taking your blood pressure places the cuff on your arm, inflates it, and then lets air out of the cuff while listening through a stethoscope to the sound of the blood passing through the artery.

Blood pressure is always recorded as two measurements. The first is the systolic pressure, which is the pressure against the blood vessel wall while the heart is contracting. The second is the diastolic pressure, which is the pressure as the heart is relaxing and filling with blood before it contracts again.

The goal for healthy adults is approximately 120 mm Hg (millimeters of mercury) systolic and 80 mm Hg diastolic. You will see the blood pressure written as systolic over diastolic, for example—120/80. If you forget which is which, remember: _d_iastolic is _d_own.

No absolute point clearly separates normal pressure from abnormal. However, blood pressure levels above 140 mm Hg systolic and/or 90 mm Hg diastolic are considered high and require medical attention. The general consensus is the lower the blood pressure the better. But if you find yourself getting dizzy when you stand up quickly, you may have hypotension, or low blood pressure, another kind of problem.

Why Should You Be Concerned About Hypertension?

Untreated or uncontrolled high blood pressure contributes, over time, to:

▲ *coronary artery disease* (chest pains—angina or heart attack)

▲ *congestive heart failure* (a condition in which the heart fails to pump properly, causing a backlog of blood that can congest the lungs and cause shortness of breath)

▲ *cerebrovascular accidents* (a stroke due to a blockage in the blood supply to the brain)

▲ *kidney disease* (the kidneys cannot properly filter wastes from the body).

If you have diabetes, you need to be particularly careful about hypertension, since it's two to three times more common in people with diabetes than in the general population. Because of your diabetes, you are at a greater risk than the general population for heart disease, stroke, and small blood vessel diseases that can damage the kidneys and the eyes. Because all of these problems are affected by hypertension, you need to do everything you can to prevent high blood pressure. If it develops, it must be treated early and aggressively.

What Should You Do If You Have Hypertension?

The National High Blood Pressure Program of the National Heart, Lung, and Blood Institute recommends the following to reduce high blood pressure:

▲ **Lose weight.** This should be the first step for people who are more than 20 pounds over their desirable body weight or who have a high percentage of body fat. Weight loss often results in a substantial drop in blood pressure. The good news, though, is that it doesn't necessarily have to be a lot of weight loss for this to happen. Research studies have reported that even 10 to 20 pounds of weight lost can be beneficial and cause an improvement in blood pressure.

▲ **Limit daily intake of sodium.** Reducing the amount of sodium you eat each day to about 2,400 milligrams (mg) will help lower your blood pressure. Research studies report a relationship between a high intake of sodium and the occurrence of high blood pressure and stroke. Blacks and persons with a family history of high blood pressure are at greatest risk for this happening. While some people are able to have normal blood pressure levels over a wide range of sodium intake, others appear to be "salt sensitive" and develop high blood pressure in response to a high sodium intake. The problem today is that no one clearly knows who is sensitive to a high sodium intake, and as a result, it is suggested that all Americans reduce sodium intake. Clearly, this will be of benefit to persons whose blood pressures do rise with sodium intake. Furthermore, there is no harm from a moderate sodium restriction.

▲ **If you drink alcohol, do so in moderation.** Limit yourself no more than 2 ounces of alcohol per day (2 ounces of liquor, 8 ounces of wine, or 24 ounces of beer).

▲ **Reduce your intake of saturated fats.** Replace them with fiber-containing carbohydrates and small amounts of unsaturated fats.

▲ **Don't smoke.** People who smoke increase their risk for coronary heart and blood vessel disease.

▲ **Get regular exercise.** It improves fitness, reduces body fat, helps control weight, and is a good way to relieve stress.

▲ **Learn to do things that are relaxing or restful for you.** Stress can aggravate high blood pressure.

In addition to these recommendations, other important suggestions for controlling high blood pressure include:

▲ **Follow medical advice in taking prescribed blood pressure medicine.** Several types of medications to control blood pressure are available and the type you use will vary, depending on certain other health problems—for example, diabetes.

▲ **When buying over-the-counter drugs, look at the ingredient list and warning statement on the label to see if sodium has been added.** Some drugs, such as antacid preparations and laxatives, can contain large amounts of sodium. If in doubt ask your pharmacist about the drug and if it is appropriate for you to use.

▲ **Avoid caffeine.** Just two or three cups of coffee each day can raise both systolic and diastolic pressure an average of 10 mm Hg or more. This increase may last up to three hours.

▲ **Have your blood pressure checked regularly.** Remember, high blood pressure often has no symptoms.

How Much Sodium Should You Eat?

When we hear the terms "salt" or "sodium," we usually think of table salt. Table salt is composed of two minerals—sodium and chloride. About one-third of the sodium in our diets comes straight from the salt shaker. So cutting down on table salt is a good way to cut down on sodium. But what about the other two-thirds? Another third comes from processed foods, and the rest from a variety of sources. Some sodium occurs naturally in foods.

By using less salt at the table and substituting alternative flavorings such as herbs, spices, and lemon juice in the preparation of foods, much can be done to reduce sodium consumption. In addition, choose lower salt foods and choose less frequently those foods to which sodium is added in processing and preservation.

Although some sodium is necessary for the body to function, we consume far more than we need. The body requires only about 220 mg of sodium per day, or the equivalent of 1/10 teaspoon of salt. (One teaspoon of salt contains 2,300 mg of sodium.) Yet the average daily intake is 4,000 to 5,000 mg of sodium—or 2 to 3 teaspoons of salt. We could easily get all the sodium we need even if we never added salt in processing or cooking food.

In general, it's recommended that we try to keep our sodium intake to less than 3,000 mg per day, or about 800 to 1,000 mg per meal. This is especially important for people who have a family history of high blood pressure.

For people who have hypertension, it is recommended they limit their sodium intake to less than 2,400 mg per day, or less than 700 mg per meal.

Everyone has individual needs. Your doctor or dietitian can help you determine what health problems you have and how much sodium you should be using. The following chart lists recommended sodium intake for various medical risks.

Recommended Sodium Intake

Health Factors	Sodium Level	Dietary Guidelines
Healthy person who wants to control sodium intake for disease prevention	3,000 milligrams per day	1) Eliminate use of table salt. 2) Seldom use foods with more than 800 milligrams of sodium per serving.
Mild hypertension Mild heart disease Mild fluid retention	2,400 milligrams per day	1) Eliminate use of table salt; use minimal amounts of salt in cooking. 2) Avoid foods containing more than 400 milligrams of sodium per serving.
Moderate to severe hypertension Kidney disease Heart disease Moderate to severe fluid retention	1,000–2,000 milligrams per day	1) Eliminate use of table salt; use minimal amounts of salt in cooking. 2) Eat only foods with less than 140 milligrams of sodium per serving.

Guidelines

▲ **Add little or no salt to foods at the table.** Remove the salt shaker from the table, and pass the pepper! Taste foods before deciding if they really need salt.

▲ **Cook with only a small amount of added salt.** When cooking pastas, vegetables, and cereals you can easily skip the salt without losing much flavor. Many recipes call for more salt than is necessary; you can use half the quantity called for and still have the same taste. In some recipes, you can leave the salt out altogether. To season stews, gravies, and soups try adding a teaspoon of prepared mustard per cup of liquid or a few hearty dashes of angostura bitters.

One caution about omitting salt in baking: Many recipes, especially those with yeast, require salt for the recipe to work.

▲ **Limit use of processed and convenience foods.** High-salt meat products (ham, bacon, sausage, cold cuts), canned soups, other canned or packaged food, and frozen entrees or dinners are other major sources of sodium.

Rinsing foods also gets rid of sodium. A one-minute rinse of 6 1/2 ounces of canned tuna will wash away about three-fourths of the sodium. Almost half the sodium can be removed from canned vegetables by rinsing for one minute and heating the vegetables in tap water instead of the canning liquid.

▲ **Experiment with herbs and spices as alternatives to salt and to salt-based condiments such as soy sauce, steak sauces, catsup, and seasoned salts.** Other flavorings to avoid include MSG (monosodium glutamate) and garlic and onion salts. Onion and garlic powders are excellent alternatives to onion and garlic salts. In place of soy sauce, steak sauce, and sea- soned salt, use lemon juice or spices such as thyme, oregano, garlic, curry, cinnamon, chili powder, or tarragon. Vinegars flavored with fresh herbs add flavor and tang to low-sodium recipes. And finally, many excellent commercial low-sodium seasonings are available including "all purpose seasonings" and herb seasonings.

When experimenting with new flavors, begin by using no more than one or two herbs or spices at a time. Start with small amounts: add ¼ teaspoon of dried herbs or 1 teaspoon of chopped fresh seasonings to soups or stews during the last hour of cooking. Adding them sooner will destroy the flavor. However, in cold dressings, dips, or marinades, add herbs and spices several hours before serving to "blend" the flavors.

As a general rule, use ¼ teaspoon of dried herbs for every four servings of food. You may want to try fresh herbs; substitute three to four times as much of the fresh herb as the dried herb. For example, if your recipe calls for 1 teaspoon of a dried herb, use 3 or 4 teaspoons of the fresh herb.

▲ **Avoid foods containing obvious amounts of salt.** This includes such foods as crackers and snack foods, pickles, olives, sauerkraut, canned soups, and so on.

▲ **Limit use of fast-foods.** Remember the sodium information provided by fast-food restaurants is based on the entire product rather than each individual component. A quick rule of thumb for fast-food dining is to limit your sodium intake at one meal to ⅓ your total sodium for the day. For example, if your daily limit is 3,000 mg, 1/3 would be 1,000 mg. Using this simple gauge can help you judge whether your fast-food dinner has too much sodium. If it does exceed the recommended amount, you need to be especially careful of your food choices during the rest of the day.

▲ **And finally, use sodium information found on food labels.** The nutrition label must tell you the milligrams of sodium per serving. Use the following guidelines to evaluate the amount of sodium listed on the label:

Look for single servings of foods that have less than 400 mg of sodium or main meal entrees with less than 800 mg of sodium.

Besides giving you the actual amount of sodium in milligrams (mg) per serving, labels may also contain descriptive terms related to sodium. A variety of terms used that are regulated by the Food and Drug Administration (FDA) and the United States Department of Agriculture (USDA).

Sodium Free. Products that contain fewer than 5 mg of sodium per serving.

Very Low Sodium. Products that contain no more than 35 mg of sodium in a serving.

Low sodium. Products that contain no more than 140 mg of sodium in a serving.

Reduced sodium. Sodium in a food product has been reduced by at least 75 percent. The product label must also include a comparison to the original product.

Unsalted, No Salt Added, Without Added Salt, Low Salt. These terms can be used only if no salt has been added to a product normally processed with salt.

How Do You Plan Meals That Are Lower in Sodium?

Exchange Lists for Meal Planning can also help you reduce sodium intake. Look for a red salt shaker or a small blue star. A red salt shaker symbol indicates foods that are high in sodium (400 mg or more of sodium per exchange). Foods that have 400 mg or more of sodium when two or more exchanges are eaten have a blue star symbol.

The following are average sodium content of commonly used foods. Remember, the general recommendation is to limit dietary sodium to less than 3,000 mg a day.

▲ List 1. Starch/Bread

Since many foods in this category are processed, the sodium content can be high. Read the label.

Breads	1 slice	110–150 mg
Hot cereals, no salt added	½ cup cooked	5 mg or less
Quick cooking and instant hot cereals	½ cup cooked	100–350 mg
Cold cereals	¾ cup	0–500 mg (check labels)
Crackers, Saltines	6	200 mg
Salt-free crackers	6	6 mg
Wheat Thins	8	120 mg
Wheat Thins, reduced salt	8	35 mg
Pasta, rice, grains (no salt added)	½ cup cooked	5 mg or less

▲ List 2. Meat and Meat Substitutes

Processed meats and main entrees can contain excessive amounts of sodium. A good rule of thumb for avoiding too much sodium is to purchase fresh meats rather than processed meats and entrees.

Cheeses, natural	1 oz	150–200 mg
Cheeses, processed	1 oz	250–350 mg
Low sodium cheese	1 oz	7–35 mg
Swiss cheese	1 oz	75 mg
Cottage cheese	½ cup	450 mg
Eggs	1	60 mg
Frankfurter	1	500 mg
Lunch meats, ham, cold cuts	1 oz	250–400 mg
Lower salt cold cuts	1 oz	200 mg
Meats, poultry, fish, fresh	3 oz	50–75 mg
Meats, fish, poultry, canned	3 oz	300–500 mg
Lower salt (50%) canned tuna	3 oz	200 mg
Peanut butter	1 tbsp.	100 mg
No salt added peanut butter	1 tbsp.	1 mg
Shellfish, fresh or frozen	3 oz	150–200 mg

▲ List 3. Vegetables

Most fresh vegetables are naturally low in sodium. Canning can add a considerable amount of sodium, so read the label. Rinsing canned vegetables significantly reduces the sodium content.

Fresh or frozen	½ cup	35 mg or less
Canned	½ cup	150–450 mg
Canned, no salt added	½ cup	35 mg or less
Tomato juice, canned	½ cup	250 mg
Vegetable (V-8) juice	½ cup	350 mg
Vegetable juice, no salt added	½ cup	35 mg

▲ List 4. Fruits

Fruits are naturally very low in sodium. Canning, freezing, or drying generally adds very little sodium.

Fruit, fruit juices	½ cup	trace–5 mg

▲ List 5. Milk

Milk naturally contains sodium. Because it is an excellent source of protein and calcium, 2 cups per day is recommended regardless of sodium restriction.

Milk	1 cup	125 mg
Buttermilk	1 cup	300 mg

▲ List 6. Fats

This category contains foods that can contain added sodium. Be sure to check the label for amounts.

Bacon	1 slice	100 mg
Margarine or butter	1 tsp.	45 mg
Margarine or butter, salt-free	1 tsp.	0–2 mg
Mayonnaise	1 tsp.	35 mg
Nuts, all kinds	¼ cup	230 mg
Salad dressings, French, Italian	1 tbsp.	150–200 mg
Salt-free salad dressings	1 tbsp.	5–10 mg

▲ Free Foods

Condiments can add the majority of sodium to prepared foods. Instead of seasoning foods with salts, try herbs and spices.

Baking soda	1 tsp.	966 mg
Bouillon	1 cube	960 mg
Catsup	1 tbsp.	155 mg
Dill pickle	1 medium	1,000 mg
Monosodium glutamate (MSG)	1 tsp.	500 mg
Salt, table salt, sea-salt, kosher, pickling	1 tsp.	2,300 mg
Lite-salt	1 tsp.	1,000 mg
Seasoned salts, onion, garlic, celery, etc.	1 tsp.	1,200–1,900 mg
Onion powder, garlic powder	1 tsp.	0 mg
Soda pop, regular or diet	12 oz.	20–70 mg
Soy sauce	1 tbsp.	1,300 mg
Lite soy sauce	1 tbsp.	600 mg
Tabasco sauce	⅛ tsp.	5 mg
Vinegars, lemon juice	any amount	0 mg
Worcestershire sauce	1 tbsp.	150 mg

There are many new "lower salt" or "no salt added" products on the market for crackers, cheeses, lunch meats, soups, canned tuna, canned vegetables, and condiments. Look for them—they will have the sodium content listed on the label.

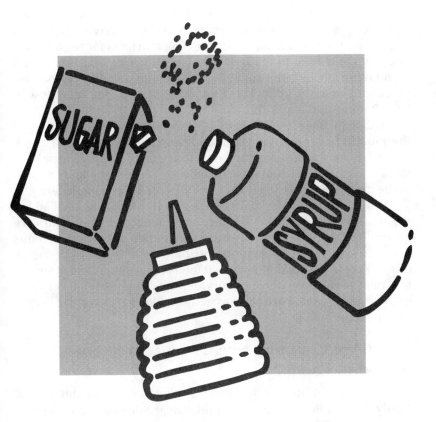

SKIP THE
ADDED SUGARS

Although sugars have not been shown to be a risk factor for any serious health problems, it still makes good sense for everyone to use added sugars in moderation. A diet with large amounts of sugars has too many calories and too few nutrients for most people and can contribute to tooth decay. The concern is not for sugars found naturally in fruits and milk, but the sugars added to foods in processing or at the table. These added sugars provide calories with few vitamins and minerals.

Although other factors also contribute to tooth decay, bacteria in the mouth can cause sugars to become acids that dissolve tooth enamel. Sugars that adhere to the teeth are more likely to cause dental cavities than those that wash off quickly. The longer sugars remain in the mouth the more likely they are to contribute to tooth decay.

People with diabetes also need to monitor their intake of added sugars. Foods that contain significant amounts of added sugars are generally high in total carbohydrate and contain significant amounts of calories as well. Both factors contribute to elevated blood glucose levels. People with diabetes can eat foods that contain added sugars but must be careful of the amounts and substitute correctly for them in their meal plans. Portion sizes of these foods as noted in Chapter 11 tend to be small.

What Are Common Sugars and Sweeteners Added to Foods?

Added sugars in the typical American diet come from soft drinks, candy, jams, jellies, syrups, and table sugar added to foods like coffee or cereal. Added sugars also come from foods such as ice cream, sweetened yogurts, chocolate milk, canned or frozen fruit with heavy syrup, and sweetened bakery products like cakes, pies, and cookies.

Sugars we are most familiar with are white sugar, brown sugar, raw sugar, corn syrup, honey, and molasses. Fructose and sorbitol are other commonly used caloric or nutritive sweeteners. But there are other sugars and sweeteners that are not as familiar. Different sugars have names that end in "ose," while other sweeteners such as sugar alcohols have names that end in "ol." The following is a brief explanation of the more common sugars and sweeteners.

Brown sugar. Made by exposing sugar crystals to a molasses syrup with natural flavoring and color or by simply adding syrup to refined white sugar in a mixture. It is 91 to 96 percent sucrose.

Corn syrup. Produced by the action of enzymes and/or acids on cornstarch. It is the liquid form of corn sugar and, when crystallized, may be called corn syrup solids or corn sweetener.

Dextrin. A sugar formed by the partial breakdown of starch.

Dextrose. Also called corn sugar. It is made from starch by the action of heat and acids, or enzymes. It is often sold for commercial use blended with regular sugar.

Fructose. Also called fruit sugar or levulose. It occurs naturally in small quantities in fruit. It has four calories per gram, as do all carbohydrates. Fructose (and sorbitol) are used in Europe as alternatives to sweeteners, such as sucrose, that contain glucose.

Crystalline fructose is a commercial sugar that is sweeter than sucrose, although its sweetness actually depends on how it's used in cooking. If used in products that are cold and acidic in nature, it tastes sweeter. If used in products that require heat, such as baking, it is usually not sweeter than sucrose. Although fructose causes a more modest increase in blood glucose levels than other sugars, it is equal in caloric value and so must be counted as part of the total caloric intake.

Fruit juice concentrate. Concentrated fruit juice that is often used to replace sucrose in jams, jellies, and other "sugar-free" products. It has little, if any, advantage over sucrose. It is not as sweet as sucrose so more is needed to provide equal sweetening power.

Galactose. Simple sugar found in lactose (milk sugar).

Glucose. The basic sugar found in the blood. It either comes from the digestion and absorption of food carbohydrates or is manufactured in the liver from other sources such as proteins. It is the form of carbohydrate that the body uses for energy.

High fructose corn syrup (HFCS). HFCS is a combination of fructose and dextrose (glucose) and is a derivative of corn. The amounts of fructose vary and many contain 42%, 55%, or 90% fructose. Glucose or dextrose comprise most of the balance. HFCS has an effect on blood glucose similar to that of sucrose. Its increased use is due to the growing market for soft drinks in which HFCS is a major ingredient.

Honey. An invert sugar formed by an enzyme from nectar gathered by bees. Its composition and flavor depend on the source of nectar. Fructose, glucose, maltose, and sucrose are among its components.

Hydrogenated starch hydrolysates (HSH). HSH is produced by a series of chemical reactions that begin with cornstarch. This produces a series of products containing mixtures of polyols (sugar alcohols). The sweetness varies from 25% to 50% of sucrose and is suitable for use in a variety of candies. It is also known as hydrogenated glucose syrup or hydrogenated sugar.

Invert sugar. A sugar formed by splitting sucrose into its component parts: glucose and fructose. This is done by an application of acids or enzymes. It is used only in liquid form and is sweeter than sucrose. Invert sugar helps prolong the freshness of baked foods and confections and is useful in preventing food shrinkage.

Lactose. The sugar found naturally in milk, which is a combination of glucose and galactose. For commercial purposes it is made from whey and skim milk. The pharmaceutical industry is a primary user of prepared lactose.

Maltose. Comes from the breakdown of starch in the malting of barley.

Mannitol. A sugar alcohol manufactured from mannose and galactose. It is half as sweet as sucrose. It is commonly used as a bulking agent in powdered foods and as a dusting agent for chewing gum. Excessive consumption may cause diarrhea.

Mannose. Comes from manna and the ivory nut, used mainly by sugar chemists.

Maple syrup. A syrup made by concentrating the sap of the sugar maple tree.

Molasses. The thick, brown syrup that is separated from raw sugar in its manufacture.

Polyols. Another name for sugar alcohols; they are synthetic products made from "ose" sugars.

Raw sugar. Tan to brown in appearance, it is a coarse, granulated solid obtained by evaporating the moisture from sugar cane juice.

Sorbitol. A sugar alcohol made commercially from glucose or dextrose, about half as sweet as sucrose. It is the most commonly used sugar alcohol. It is readily converted to fructose and is similarly used by the body. One of the major problems with sorbitol is that it may cause diarrhea in some people. Also, many products sweetened with sorbitol contain as many or more calories than the product they are replacing because of the added fat used to dissolve the sorbitol and give the food a creamy texture.

Sorghum. Syrup from the sweet juice of the sorghum grain.

Sucrose. Crystals from cane or beet sugars. It is composed of two simple sugars, glucose and fructose. Sucrose is about 99.9 percent pure and sold either granulated, cubed, or powdered.

Turbinado sugar. Sometimes viewed erroneously as raw sugar. It actually has to go through a refining process to remove impurities and most of the molasses. It is produced by separating raw sugar crystals and washing them with steam.

Xylitol. A sugar alcohol manufactured from xylose (wood sugar from part of the birch tree). Its sweetness is about equal to sucrose.

What Are High-Intensity Sweeteners?

High-intensity sweeteners are also called nonnutritive or low- or non-caloric sweeteners. They are intensely sweet, so only very small amounts of them are needed to sweeten food products. Examples are saccharin, aspartame, acesulfame-K, sucralose, cyclamates, and alitame. Several are not currently approved for use in the United States by the Food and Drug Administration (FDA). They are primarily alternatives to sucrose. Although some of these products may contribute calories, they are used in such small quantities that they do not make a significant contribution to caloric intake.

A term to be familiar with is *accepted daily intake (ADI)*. The ADI is the amount of a food additive that is determined by the FDA to be safe for humans to consume on a daily basis over a lifetime without adverse effects. This is about 1/100 of the amount tested and shown to have no toxic effects in animals. The ADI is reported as an amount per kilogram (2.2 pounds equals 1 kg) of body weight. For example, 50 mg/kg is the ADI for aspartame. For a 150-pound (70 kg) person, this represents twenty 12-oz cans of diet soft drinks sweetened with aspartame or 97 packets of Equal, and for a 50-pound (45 kg) child, seven diet soft drinks or 32 packets of Equal to reach ADI levels. As you can see, the ADI includes a very generous safety factor.

A variety of sweeteners allows for more low-calorie food products. And with several alternative sweeteners available, each can be used in the applications for which it is best suited. Sweetener limitations can also be minimized by combining them. The following high-intensity sweeteners are currently available for use in the United States:

Saccharin. Although saccharin has been used for about 80 years, in 1977 it was designated by the FDA as a possible cancer-causing agent. A two-generation male rat study showed a probability of inducing cancer in second-generation rats with an intake of saccharin that was equivalent to about 800 cans of diet soda a day. However, there is no evidence to suggest it causes cancer in humans. In December 1991, the FDA withdrew its 1977 proposal to ban saccharin. However, the saccharin warning must still remain on labels.

Aspartame. Aspartame is a combination of two amino acids (aspartic acid and phenylalanine) that when combined are intensely sweet. It is marketed as a tabletop sweetener called Equal®. Under the brand name of NutraSweet®, aspartame is used in a variety of food products. Beginning in 1993 aspartame will have other brand names. Before it was approved for use in foods, aspartame underwent more than 100 scientific studies during the past 20 years. According to the FDA, "few compounds have withstood such detailed testing and repeated close scrutiny."

The only documented harm from aspartame affects people with a very rare inherited disease called phenylketonuria (PKU). This is why a warning to people with PKU appears on all foods containing Equal or NutraSweet.

Acesulfame-K. Acesulfame-K is a manmade sweetener with a high degree of stability when exposed to heat. It is marketed under the brand name of Sunette®, as SweetOne®, or Swiss Sweet™ tabletop sweeteners. Acesulfame-K has been reviewed and determined to be safe by regulatory authorities in more than 20 countries. Its safety is supported by more than 90 studies conducted over 15 years.

Sucralose. Approved for use in Canada, sucralose is the first sugar substitute made from sugar. It's the only substitute to combine the taste of sugar with stability in processed foods and beverages. It has no calories and can be used virtually anywhere sugar can be used, including cooking and baking. Sucralose retains sweetness over long storage periods and at elevated temperatures. Extensive studies have been conducted and evaluated to show and support that sucralose is safe for humans to use.

Cyclamate. In 1973 cyclamates were removed from the market, principally on the basis of one experiment when its use at a very high dose was related to the development of bladder tumors in rats . However, 75 subsequent studies have failed to demonstrate that cyclamate causes cancer. The FDA is currently reviewing a petition for reapproval.

Alitame. Alitame is formed from the amino acids aspartic acid and alanine. It is also stable at high temperatures and would be suitable for use in a wide variety of products such as beverages, tabletop sweeteners, frozen desserts, and baked goods. Alitame has been shown to be safe in more than 15 studies, but as part of the food additive process, the FDA requested that an animal study on alitame be repeated. This additional study is expected to delay approval in the United States to the mid-1990s.

Guidelines

Although humans have no inborn craving or urge for fat or salt, we naturally like sweetness. Animals too, with the exception of cats, have a "sweet tooth." However, many humans have fed their "sweet tooth" so well that they crave unhealthy levels of sugar.

The key is to reduce your intake of refined (table sugar) and added sugars (used in baked goods or in the manufacturing process of many foods). These sugars currently contribute 25 percent of the average American's total calories, or the equivalent of 12 table-spoons of sugar daily. An appropriate goal is to reduce sugar to approximately 10 percent of the total energy intake.

▲ **Eat fruits, low-fat dairy products, or breads for dessert.** Eat baked products with ingredients such as oatmeal, whole wheat flour, raisins, pumpkin, zucchini, or carrots instead of eating cakes, cookies, or pies. Dessert powders such as Jello are 85 percent sugar and 10 percent gelatin plus factory made flavoring and color.

▲ **Avoid buying sweet snacks to have in the house.** Cut back on commercial baked goods such as pastries, sweet rolls, and cookies, which are the second biggest source of sugar after soft drinks. One candy bar has as much sugar as ½ pound of apples. An average serving of pancake syrup is ¼ cup. This is as much sugar as found in four to five apples or oranges.

▲ **Substitute fruit juices, skim milk, and water for soft drinks.** The soft drink industry is the largest single source of sugar in the diet. The sugar in one 12-ounce can of cola supplies 145 calories or the equivalent of nine to ten teaspoons of sugar.

▲ **Reduce the amount of sugar called for in recipes.** Sugars and other sweeteners add flavor, color, tenderness, and crispness in baked products. In many recipes, however, you can reduce the sugar called for by at least ½ to ⅓ without affecting the quality of the product. A helpful guideline: use no more than ¼ cup of added sweetener (sugar, honey, molasses, and so on) per one cup of flour. Every ¼ cup of sugar adds close to 200 empty calories to your recipes. Vanilla, cinnamon, and nutmeg all give the illusion of sweetness without adding calories.

Use The Following Guidelines When Sweetening Without Sugar

1. Aspartame should not be added before cooking in the oven or on the range, because the heat may cause it to lose its sweetness. It may be added to foods after the cooking process.

2. When using fructose in cooking or baking, use one third less fructose than the amount of sugar called for in the recipe. Since fructose contains calories and carbohydrate, foods with fructose in them need to be counted in the meal plan.

3. Liquid non-caloric sweeteners can be added directly to the mixture.

4. Non-caloric sweetening tablets may be crushed and stirred into a liquid mixture, or they may be dissolved first in a small amount of liquid called for in the recipe and then added to the rest of the mixture.

5. Granulated sweeteners, including NutraSweet Spoonful, may be added in the same way sugar would be added to cold or non-baked recipes.

6. In cooking with saccharin, it is generally best, if possible, to add the sweetening agent toward the end of the cooking cycle or immediately afterwards, because saccharin tends to lose its sweetening power after exposure to high temperatures or to extended lower cooking temperatures (as in baking); heat increases the bitter flavor of saccharin.

7. Acesulfame-K is stable to heat and therefore can be used in cooking and baking. For best results use recipes developed for use with SweetOne or experiment by substituting half the sugar called for with the equivalent amount of SweetOne.

8. Call or write manufacturers (addresses are on the label) for recipes especially made for their particular sugar substitute.

▲

A Handy Guide to Sweetening without Sugar

Type of Sweetener and Brand Name	Major Sweetening Ingredient	Sweetness Compared to Sugar Amt. Sweetener = Amt. Sugar	Manufacturer's Suggested Uses
High Intensity Sweeteners			
EQUAL, packets or tablets	Aspartame	1 packet = 2 tsp. 1 tablet = 1 tsp.	Table use, added to cold/hot foods (if added after cooking).
NUTRASWEET SPOONFUL	Aspartame	1 tsp. = 1 tsp.	Table use, added to cold or non-baked recipes
SPRINKLE SWEET, packets	Saccharin	1 packet = 2 tsp.	Baking, cooking, and table use.
SUGAR TWIN, regular and brown sugar replacement, powder and packets	Saccharin	1 tsp. = 1 tsp. 1 Tbsp. = 1 Tbsp. 1 cup = 1 cup 1 packet = 2 tsp.	Baking, cooking, and table use.

Type of Sweetener and Brand Name	Major Sweetening Ingredien	Sweetness Compared to Sugar Amt. Sweetener = Amt. Sugar	Manufacturer's Suggested Uses
SWEET 10 liquid	Saccharin	⅛ tsp. (10 drops)=1 tsp. ⅜ tsp. = 1 Tbsp. 2 Tbsp. = 1 cup	Table use and in cooking.
SWEET MATE	Aspartame	1 packet = 2 tsp.	Table use and added to cold or hot foods (if added after cooking).
SWEET 'N' LOW regular and brown sugar replacement, powder and packets	Saccharin	1 tsp. = ¼ cup 1⅓ tsp. = ⅓ cup 2 tsp. = ½ cup 4 tsp. = 1 cup 1 packet = 2 tsp.	Baking, cooking, canning, and table use.
SWEET ONE	Acesulfame-K	1 packet = 2 tsp. 3 packets = ¼ cup 4 packets = ⅓ cup 6 packets = ½ cup 12 packets = 1 cup	Table use, baking, and cooking.
SWISS SWEET	Acesulfame-K	1 packet = 2 tsp.	Table use, baking and cooking.
Nutritive Sweeteners Fructose, powder and packets	Fructose	1 tsp. = 12 calories and 3 grams carbohydrate 1 packet = 1 tsp. fructose powder	Table use and in cooking; tastes sweeter in cold foods.

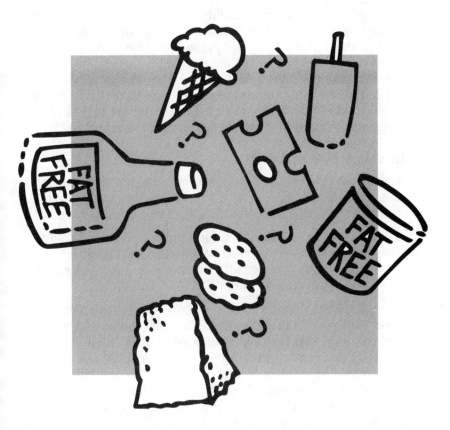

FAT SUBSTITUTES—
PROBLEMS OR A
PANACEA?

Sugar substitutes have been on the market since the early 1950s. But despite their availability, sugar consumption has not decreased. In fact, since 1965 sugar consumption has risen by 14 percent to about 130 pounds per person per year while the use of artificial sweeteners has more than doubled.

So what about fat substitutes? Can they be more useful in reducing fat and calorie intake than sugar substitutes have been in reducing sugar intake? Or will consumers simply eat more of these foods using the justification that they do not contain much fat.

What Are Fat Substitutes?

Ingredients: cultured sour cream, skim milk, whey protein concentrate, water, food starch-modified, lactic acid, maltodextrin, cellulose gum, potassium sorbate (a preservative), agar, vitamin A palmitate.

Ingredients: water, soybean oil, sugar, vinegar, food starch-modified, salt, starch, cellulose gel (microcrystalline cellulose), sodium caseinate, mustard flour, egg white, xanthan gum, spice, paprika, natural flavor, beta carotene (color).

Can you identify the fat substitutes in the above two ingredient listings? The first lists the ingredients in a light sour cream and the second the ingredients in light reduced-calorie salad dressing. Chances are you can't, yet the first product may have five ingredients that could be used as fat substitutes and the second product three. In the first product, whey protein concentrate, food starch-modified, maltodextrin, cellulose gum, and agar can all play a role as a fat substitute and in the second, food starch-modified, cellulose gel (microcrystalline cellulose), and xanthan gum may be fat substitutes.

In response to consumers' concerns about the amount of fat and calories they eat, the food industry is researching replacements for fat. Many of them are already being used in food products and more are on the drawing board or being petitioned to the FDA for approval for use.

Fat replacements can be grouped according to what they are made from—carbohydrate, protein, or fat—or according to the number of calories they contribute to the diet. For instance, some are calorie-reduced substitutes while others are calorie-free substitutes. The products used today fall into the category of being calorie-reduced.

Calorie-reduced substitutes are made by substituting lower-calorie carbohydrates and protein for fat. They are digested and absorbed normally and provide one to four calories per gram in comparison to nine from fat. Fat substitutes currently in use fall into the category the FDA calls GRAS (Generally Recognized as Safe). Because they are carbohydrate- or protein-based and have long been used in foods for other purposes, safety studies are not required.

Substituting Carbohydrates for Fat

For more than a decade, some carbohydrates have been used to partially or totally replace fats or oils in a wide variety of food products. The carbohydrate-based fat replacements include dextrins, maltodextrins, modified food starches, polydextrose, cellulose, and gums. Dextrins and modified food starches are bland, nonsweet carbohydrates that have water added and as a result form gels that mimic the texture and mouth-feel of fat. They can be derived from wheat, potato, corn, tapioca, rice, or combined starches.

Polydextrose is a nonsweet starch made from dextrose and small amounts of sorbitol and citric acid. It was initially developed as a bulking agent for non-nutritive sweeteners but can also replace up to one-half of the fat in a product. Microcrystalline cellulose is made from purified wood pulp processed to form a gel. It can replace a percentage of fat in salad dressings and frozen desserts.

Gums such as xanthane gum, guar gum, carageenans, and water can also be used to stabilize the consistency of foods in place of fat. Algins from kelp are also used as stabilizers in pourable salad dressings. They are not digested so the calories are negligible.

Proteins Used as Fat Substitutes

The NutraSweet Company, manufacturer of aspartame, is also developing a fat substitute, Simplesse®. It is made from all-natural protein, either egg whites or milk protein, by a process called microparticulation. By this process, protein is heated and blended to create very, very small round particles. These particles flow over the tongue to create a rich, creamy taste similar to fat. It supplies 1⅓ calories per gram compared to 9 calories per gram from fat. It can't be used in products that will be heated, such as oils used for frying or baking. The heat would cause the protein to gel and lose its creamy consistency.

Microparticulation does not change the protein in any way uncommon to cooking. The body digests and absorbs Simplesse like any other protein. Products made with Simplesse should, therefore, be safe for anyone without sensitivities to egg or milk products. The FDA declared Simplesse as GRAS and safety studies were not required.

Simple Pleasures is a frozen dessert made with Simplesse. In the chart below you can see that you save some calories in these products, but if it makes people who eat products made with fat substitutes feel free to eat more other high-fat foods, or eat more fat-free double-dip ice cream cones, they won't be saving many calories.

| | Per 4 ounce serving | |
	Grams of fat	Calories
Simple Pleasure	1	120
Regular ice cream	7	135
Premium ice cream	19	276

Fat Substitutes Made from Fats or Oils

Olestra is an example of a calorie-free fat replacement. It is a combination of sugar and oils brought together by a process combining high temperature and pressure. Because the resulting molecule has a larger size and shape, the body's digestive enzymes are unable to break it down, and it cannot be absorbed into the bloodstream and converted to calories. However, it has the same taste and cooking properties as regular oils and fats. Olestra can be used wherever fats are used, even in high temperature cooking such as baking and deep frying. The food company developing olestra is petitioning the FDA to begin approving use of olestra in snacks at 100% replacement of fat and is seeking approval to market fat-free potato chips, corn chips, and snacks of this type.

Caprenin is a fat substitute made from fat that is currently being used in food products. It has properties similar to those of cocoa butter and so is used in candies and in confectionery coatings for nuts, fruits, cookies, and so on. Unlike other fats that supply nine calories per gram, caprenin provides five calories per gram. Although it can lower fat content from 11 to 8 grams and calories from 280 to 190 in a candy bar, the candy bar still contains fat and contributes calories to the diet.

Other calorie-free substitutes made from fats have very long names and are usually abbreviated with the use of initials. Some of them are listed in the chart at the end of this chapter. None of these products has yet been approved by the FDA.

Fat-Free or Fat-Reduced Versions of Traditional Foods

Instead of developing fat substitutes, some food companies are developing fat-free or fat-reduced foods. These foods have less than 1 gram of fat per serving, yet they maintain desirable product characteristics such as taste and texture. To date, fat-free versions of foods have been introduced in seven food categories: processed cheese, salad dressings, yogurt, frozen yogurt, frozen desserts, frozen dessert bars, and fat-free baked goods such as pastries, cookies, cakes, and so on.

Guidelines

Fat replacements are not a "free ride." They will only be used in a limited number of food products and often only as partial replacement for fat. The substitutes won't cure the problem you can cause yourself at the dinner table. A balanced diet including a variety of foods is still essential.

You still need to watch the amount you eat. For example, a one-ounce serving (about two tablespoons) of light sour cream has 40 calories compared to 62 calories from regular sour cream and 2 grams of fat rather than 6. A one tablespoon serving of light reduced-calorie salad dressing has 45 calories compared to 70 calories from regular salad dressing and 4 grams of fat instead of 7.

If sugar and fat substitutes are used reasonably in the diet, they have the potential to help persons reduce fat, sugar, and calories in the diet. However, if they destroy the incentive for people to continue to eat well, and instead focus attention on such foods as ice cream, cookies, potato chips, and other snack foods that are not nutritionally good for them, they won't be particularly helpful.

Whether the taste is acceptable and whether they satisfy hunger are other issues, but the bottom line is that food substitutes can't be viewed as a magic potion for weight control or healthful eating. How helpful they are depends on how you use them.

The following chart lists fat replacements being used in food products and that are under development. Because these products are designed for use by different food processing companies, they have not been developed with consumer brand names. Ingredients will appear on the labels under their common or usual names such as dextrins, maltodextrins, modified food starches. You may not recognize them as a fat substitute. Column one lists the common name with examples of brand names used by the company to market these products to other food companies. Column two lists terms for the fat substitute that will appear on the label ingredient list and column three lists some of the food products the fat substitutes are used in.

Fat Replacements

Carbohydrate-Based Fat Replacement	How Product is Listed on Ingredient Label	Uses
Dextrins N-Oil Nutri C Oatrim	Wheat, potato, corn, tapioca dextrin Beta-glucan amylodextrin	Salad dressings, puddings, spreads, dairy-type products, frozen desserts
Maltodextrins Maltrin Paselli SA2 Star-Dri	Maltodextrins, corn syrup solids, hydrolyzed corn starch, glucose polymers Potato maltodextrin	Baked goods, dairy products, salad dressings, spreads, sauces, frostings and fillings, frozen desserts, processed meats
Modified Food Starch Sta-Slim 143 Ultra-Freeze 400 Stellar	Modified food starch, vegetable protein, corn syrup Food starch modified	Processed meats, salad dressings, baked goods, fillings and frostings, sauces, condiments, frozen desserts, dairy products

Carbohydrate-Based Fat Replacement	How Product is Listed on Ingredient Label	Uses
Polydextrose Litesse	Polydextrose	Baked goods, chewing gum, confections, salad dressings, frozen dairy desserts, gelatins, puddings
Cellulose Avicel	Microcrystalline cellulose	Dairy-type products, sauces, frozen desserts, salad dressings
Gums	Xanthan gum, guar gum, locust bean gum, gum arabic carrageenan	Reduced calorie and fat-free salad dressings, processed meats

Protein-Based Fat Replacements	How Product is Listed on Ingredient Label	Uses
Microparticulated Protein Simplesse	Microparticulated egg white and milk protein, protein concentrate	Dairy-type products (ice cream, butter, sour cream, cheese, yogurt), salad dressings, margarines, mayonnaise-type products. Frozen desserts and baked goods
Other Protein Blends Trailblazer Finese	Same as above	Same as above

Fat-Based Fat Replacers	How Product is Listed on Ingredient Label	Uses
Caprenin	Caprenin	Soft candies, confectionery coatings for nuts and fruits, cookies
Sucrose Polyesters Olestra*	Not yet determined	Home cooking oils and shortenings, commercial frying and snack foods
Lipid (Fat/Oil) Analogs DDM*	Not yet determined	Chips, mayonnaise- and margarine-type products
EPG*	Not yet determined	Formulated products, baking and frying
TATCA*	Not yet determined	Margarine and mayonnaise-type products

*Will require FDA approval.

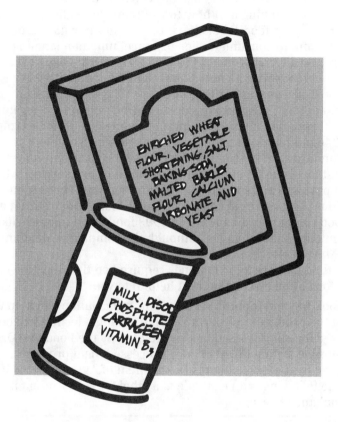

FOOD LABELS—
TRYING TO END
CONFUSION

Labels can help you decide which foods are appropriate to use in meal planning and how to use them correctly. New regulations regarding food labels have made the information on labels more helpful to consumers. For instance, nutrition labeling is now required on all food products (except for restaurant and delicatessen foods and foods with no nutritional significance such as spices) and must be based on standard serving sizes. These serving sizes are the amount of food "customarily consumed" at one time. They must be listed in common household and metric measures, for example, 1 cup, 240 milliliters, and unless a single-serving container is double the standard size, the container must be labeled as only one serving. For instance, one 12-ounce can of soda is now one serving, whereas in the past ½ of a 12-ounce can was one serving. These regulations should make it easier to compare similar food products from different food companies. Beginning in 1993 food companies are likely to start making label changes, although the compliance deadline isn't until May 1994.

Although more information is required on the label, the following information can be the most helpful to you:

▲ **Look for nutritional labeling.** This information can help you fit the product into your meal plan. A single format will be used for all processed foods regulated by the Food and Drug Administration (FDA) and for processed meat products regulated by the United States Department of Agriculture (USDA). The following is an example of a label for ready-to-eat macaroni and cheese:

Nutrition facts		
Serving size ½ cup (114g)		
Servings per container 4		
Amount per serving		
Calories 260 Calories from fat 120		
		% Daily Value*
Total Fat 13g		20%
Saturated Fat 5g		25%
Cholesterol 30 mg		10%
Sodium 660g		28%
Total Carbohydrate 31 g		11%
Sugars 5g		
Dietary Fiber 0g		0%
Protein 5g		
Vitamin A 4%	Vitamin C 2%	
Calcium 15%	Iron 4%	

*Percent (%) of a Daily Value are based on a 2,000 calorie diet. Your Daily Values may vary higher or lower depending on your calorie needs:

Nutrient	2,000 Calories	2,500 Calories
Total Fat	Less than 65g	80g
Sat. Fat	Less than 20g	25g
Cholesterol	Less than 300mg	300mg
Sodium	Less than 2,400mg	2,400mg
Total Carbohydrate	300g	375g
Fiber	25g	30g

1g Fat = 9 calories
1g Carbohydrate = 4 calories
1g Protein = 4 calories

▲ **Look at the list of ingredients.** They will tell you what a product contains and will help you decide whether you should use a particular product.

▲ **Look at the descriptive terms and health claims on the label.** There are now uniform definitions that food producers and marketers must use for descriptive terms such as light, low fat, low sodium, and so forth. There are also specific guidelines for health claims. For example, health claims are only allowed relating calcium to osteoporosis, sodium to hypertension, and fat to heart disease and cancer. No other claims linking foods to a health problem or chronic disease can be made on labels.

Your First Clue: Nutrition Labeling

Look at the calories, grams of total fat, total carbohydrate, and protein listed on the nutrition label. Although more information is required, this information based on the serving size can be translated into exchanges. At the end of the chapter the steps to do this are explained.

Knowing the number of calories per serving can be helpful in deciding how to fit a product into your meal plan. If a food contains less than 20 calories per serving, it may be used as a free food either at mealtime or at snacktime. However, free foods, if they contain calories, should be limited to one per meal or not more than three per day for a total of 50 to 60 calories.

Nutrition information on food labels will be put into the context of sample daily diet for 2,000 calories and 65 grams of fat. Instead of Recommended Daily Allowances, labels will list percentages of Daily Values calculated using the 2,000 calorie diet. However, the new labels will also contain daily allotments of fat and other nutrients based on a 2,500 calorie diet. The statement, "Your Daily Values may vary higher or lower depending on your calorie needs," appearing on labels recognizes that people of different ages, activity levels, and gender have different calorie needs.

Percentages can be misleading. It is much more helpful to know the actual amount in weight (grams) contained in a product than the percentage of calories from fat, saturated or unsaturated fats, or from sugar. For example, an ounce of a meat product may have 62 percent of its calories from fat but still contain only 5 grams of fat. Or a glass of cola (because it is primarily water) may have a lower percentage of sugar than a bouillon cube but actually contain significantly more sugar.

Milligrams of sodium in a serving size is also useful information. As mentioned in Chapter 24, look for single servings of foods with less than 400 mg of sodium and entire meals with less than 800 mg. Milligrams of cholesterol, grams of saturated fat, sugars and dietary fiber, and the amounts of vitamins A and C, calcium, and iron may also be useful information for you.

Your Second Clue: Ingredient Listing

Also look at the ingredient listing; ingredients must be listed in descending order according to the percentage of weight they contribute to the total product. A change in labeling laws now requires that on the ingredient listing sweeteners must be grouped together in parentheses after the word "sweeteners," in descending order of predominance. For example, the ingredient listing on raspberry jam is currently: corn syrup, raspberries, sugar, fruit pectin, citric acid. Under the new labeling guidelines, the ingredient listing would be the following: sweeteners (corn syrup, sugar), raspberries, fruit pectin, citric acid.

Be aware of ingredients that are high in saturated fat. Some of these are: animal fat, bacon, beef fat, or chicken fat; butter; cocoa butter or chocolate; coconut or coconut oil; palm or palm kernel oil; hardened or hydrogenated shortenings, fats, or oil; and lard. Again look at the total grams of fat in the serving size to determine if these ingredients are contained in significant amounts.

If you have been advised to limit your sodium intake, be on the lookout for the following high sodium ingredients: bouillon, brine (salt and water), broth, monosodium glutamate (MSG), salt or sodium chloride, and soy sauce.

Third Clue: Descriptive Terms

Besides the health claims listed above labels also contain descriptors and nutrient content claims. These are now much better regulated than in the past. Calories, sodium, total fat, saturated fat, cholesterol, and sugars now have specific guidelines they must meet in order to claim they are "free" of the nutrient; "low," "reduced," or have "less" of the nutrient; or claim to contain "more"; be a "source" or be a "good source"; or "high," "rich in," or "major source of." Furthermore, terms such as "light"/"lite" and "modified" are also defined. For example, a food can be described as "light" or "lite" only if it has 50 percent less fat than the food to which it is compared. The word "more" can be used only if a food product contains 10 percent more of a given ingredient than other foods of the same type.

New regulations will allow manufacturers to produce healthier versions of some products and still use the recognized name, such as "low-fat ice cream," if the product meets the definition of "low fat." In the past if products did not meet the butterfat guidelines for products such as ice cream, cheese, and sour cream, they could not do this. These products would be labeled as an "imitation" or "substitute" or have a new name such as "frozen dietary dessert" or "cheese food."

All of the changes should help end the confusion when it comes to deciphering food labels.

Using Nutritional Labeling

In order to use the information from the nutrition label effectively, you must first understand the basis for grouping foods into exchange lists. The indicated amount of each food in a single list contains approximately the same number of calories and grams of carbohydrate, protein, and fat.

By looking at the nutrition information on the label you can estimate how many exchanges are in a serving of a food and how to include it in your meal plan. Pay particular attention to the grams of carbohydrate, protein, and fat, although the grams do not need to be exactly equal to the number in the exchanges. In most meal plans, variations of a few calories or grams of carbohydrate, protein, or fat are not significant.

Use the following table and example to convert information from a label to the exchange system.

▲

Amounts of Nutrients in Food Exchanges

Exchange	Calories	Carbohydrate	Protein	Fat
1 starch/bread	80	15 gm	3 gm	trace
1 lean meat	55	–	7 gm	3 gm
1 medium-fat meat	75	–	7 gm	5 gm
1 high-fat meat	100	–	7 gm	8 gm
1 vegetable	25	5 gm	2 gm	–
1 fruit	60	15 gm	–	–
1 milk (skim)	90	12 gm	8 gm	trace
1 fat	45	–	–	5 gm

Steps for Converting Nutritional Labeling to Exchanges

The following label is from a 10-oz box of frozen pizza.

Nutritional Information Per Serving
Serving size ....½ pizza (5 oz)
Servings per container...........................2
Calories...350
Protein..17 gm
Carbohydrate ....33 gm
Fat ....16 gm

To make it easier to convert label information to the exchange system, follow these steps:

1. Check the label for the information you need to convert to the exchange system. You need:

Serving size ....½ pizza (5 oz)
Calories...350
Protein..17 gm
Carbohydrate ....33 gm

2. Check the serving size. Is this a reasonable size for your use?

3. Compare the label information with the carbohydrate, protein, fat, and calories on the exchange table. First, look at the amount and source of carbohydrate in the food product. In this case, you'll be converting the carbohydrate to starch/bread exchanges. Note in the exchange table that 15 gm of carbohydrate and 3 gm of protein equal 1 starch/bread exchange. This means that 30 gm of carbohydrate plus 6 gm of the protein in your pizza serving equal 2 starch/bread exchanges.

	Carbohydrate	Protein	Fat
½ pizza	33 gm	17 gm	16 gm
2 starch/bread exchanges	30 gm	6 gm	–

4. Next, subtract the grams of protein you used in figuring the starch/bread exchanges from the total amount of protein in the serving size. Then convert the remaining grams of protein to meat exchanges. Use the medium-fat meat exchange values from the exchange table.

	Carbohydrate	Protein	Fat
½ pizza	33 gm	17 gm	16 gm
2 starch/bread exchanges	30 gm	– 6 gm	–
		11 gm	16 gm
2 medium-fat meat exchanges		14 gm	10 gm

5. Next, subtract the grams of fat in the meat exchanges from the fat contained in the serving size. Then convert the remaining grams of fat to fat exchanges.

	Carbohydrate	Protein	Fat
½ pizza	33 gm	17 gm	16 gm
2 starch/bread exchanges	30 gm	– 6 gm	–
		11 gm	16 gm
2 medium-fat meat exchanges		14 gm	– 10 gm
			6 gm
1 fat exchange			5 gm

6. If you eat ½ of this 10-oz pizza, you use the following exchanges from your meal plan: 2 starch/bread, 2 medium-fat meat, 1 fat

7. Final check:

	Carbohydrate	Protein	Fat	Calories
½ pizza	*33 gm*	*17 gm*	*16 gm*	*350*
Exchanges:				
2 starch/bread,	*30 gm*	6 gm		*160*
2 medium-fat meat,		+<u>14 gm</u>	10 gm	*150*
1 fat		20 gm	+<u>5 gm</u>	<u>45</u>
			15 gm	355

8. If the difference between the grams per serving and the grams accounted for by the exchange system is less than half of an exchange, you do not need to count those extra grams.

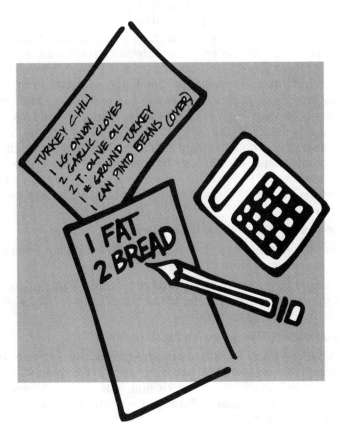

CALCULATING EXCHANGES FROM YOUR FAVORITE RECIPES

If you have favorite recipes that you enjoy or that you have modified and make often, you may wish to know how many exchanges are in a serving of your recipe so you can fit it into your meal plan. You can use two methods to convert your recipes to exchanges. Both use the information from the table Commonly Used Baking and Cooking Ingredients, which appears later in this chapter. The first way to do this is to use the exchange values of the ingredients in your recipe and divide the total exchanges by the number of servings in the recipe. The second way to do this is to write down the carbohydrate, protein, and fat listed for the ingredients in your recipe; divide each by the number of servings in the recipe; and convert the results into exchanges using the steps as outlined in Chapter 27 for converting food labeling information into exchanges.

For the first method follow these steps:

1. List all ingredients in the recipe and their amounts. Form 1 at the end of this chapter can be used to do this.
2. Convert each ingredient into the number of appropriate exchanges it provides. Refer to the table Commonly Used Baking and Cooking Ingredients.
3. Total each exchange group for the entire recipe.
4. Divide the total exchanges by the number of servings in the recipe. You can round off these numbers to the nearest one-half exchange. Anything less than one-half does not need to be counted. Form 2 is an example of a recipe that has been converted into exchanges.

For the second method follow these steps:

1. List all ingredients in the recipe and their amounts.
2. List the amount of carbohydrate, protein, and fat in each ingredient. Use the values from the table Commonly Used Baking and Cooking Ingredients.
3. Total the grams of carbohydrate, protein, and fat for the entire recipe.
4. Divide the grams of carbohydrate, protein, and fat by the number of servings in the recipe. Follow the steps for converting the results to exchanges as listed on pages 252 to 254.

COMMONLY USED BAKING
▲ AND COOKING INGREDIENTS ▲

FOOD	QTY.	CARBO-HYDRATE (gm)	PROTEIN (gm)	FAT (gm)	EXCHANGES
Starches:					
Biscuit mix	½ cup	37	4	8	2½ starch/bread 1 fat
Bread crumbs, dry	1 cup	65	11	4	4 starch/bread
Graham cracker crumbs	1 cup	90	8	14	6 starch/bread 2 fat
Chow mein noodles	½ cup	17	3	8	1 starch/bread 1½ fat
Cornmeal, uncooked	1 cup	117	11	5	7½ starch/bread
Cornstarch	2 Tbsp.	14	–	–	1 starch/bread
Cream soup, undiluted	1 can, 10¾ oz	22	5	19	1½ starch/bread 3½ fat
Flour					
all-purpose	1 cup	87	11	1	6 starch/bread
whole wheat	1 cup	80	16	2	5 starch/bread
rye	1 cup	66	10	2	4½ starch/bread
cake, sifted	1 cup	79	8	1	5 starch/bread
Macaroni					
uncooked, 3½ oz	1 cup	79	7	trace	5 starch/bread
cooked	1 cup	41	7	1	3 starch/bread
Noodles, egg					
uncooked, 2½ oz	1 cup	59	7	1	4 starch/bread
cooked	1 cup	40	8	3	2½ starch/bread
Oatmeal, uncooked	1 cup	54	15	6	3½ starch/bread 1 fat
Rice, white & brown					
uncooked	¼ cup	39	3	–	2½ starch/bread
cooked	1 cup	36	3	1	2½ starch/bread
wild, uncooked	¼ cup	21	4	–	1½ starch/bread
long grain, instant, dry	¼ cup	26	2	–	2 starch/bread
long grain, instant cooked	1 cup	40	4	–	2½ starch/bread
Spaghetti					
uncooked, 3½ oz.	1 cup	79	7	trace	5 starch/bread
cooked	1 cup	41	7	1	2½ starch/bread

FOOD	QTY.	CARBO-HYDRATE (gm)	PROTEIN (gm)	FAT (gm)	EXCHANGES
Wheat germ, 1 oz.	¼ cup	13	9	3	1 starch/bread 1 lean meat
Dairy Products:					
Butter or margarine	¼ cup, ½ stick	–	–	49	10 fat
	½ cup, 1 stick	–	–	98	20 fat
Cheese					
cheddar, shredded	1 cup	2	29	37	4 high fat meat 1 fat
cream	4 oz.	3	8	40	1 high fat meat 6 fat
mozzarella, part- skim, shredded	1 cup	3	28	18	4 med. fat meat
Parmesan, grated	¼ cup	1	8	6	1 med. fat meat
Cream					
half and half	½ cup	5	3	14	3 fat
sour	½ cup	4	3	20	5 fat
heavy, unwhipped	¼ cup	2	1	22	4 fat
heavy, whipped	½ cup	2	1	22	4 fat
Egg					
whole	1 medium	–	6	6	1 med.fat.meat
yolk	1 medium	–	3	5	1 fat
Milk					
condensed, sweetened	⅓ cup	54	8	9	1 skim milk 3 fruit 2 fat
evaporated, whole	½ cup	12	8	10	1 skim milk 2 fat
evaporated, skim	½ cup	14	9	–	1 skim milk
nonfat dry, instant	1 cup	31	21	–	2½ skim milk
Yogurt					
plain, nonfat	1 cup	17	12	–	1 skim milk
Fats, Oils, Chocolate, Cocoa:					
Chocolate, bitter unsweetened	1 oz	7	4	16	½ starch/bread 3 fat
Chocolate flavored syrup	2 Tbsp.	17	1	1	1 fruit
Chocolate chips	1 cup	105	8	48	7 fruit 10 fat
Carob powder	1 cup	113	6	2	7½ starch/bread

FOOD	QTY.	CARBO-HYDRATE (gm)	PROTEIN (gm)	FAT (gm)	EXCHANGES
Cocoa powder	¼ cup	16	6	2	1 starch/bread
Mayonnaise	½ cup	1	1	88	17½ fat
Mayonnaise-type salad dressing	½ cup	14	1	55	1 starch/bread 11 fat
Olives, sliced	½ cup	2	1	15	3 fat
Shortening	½ cup	–	–	111	22 fat
Vegetable oil	½ cup	–	–	111	22 fat
Fruits and Vegetables:					
Barbecue sauce	3 Tbsp.	15	–	1	1 fruit
Catsup	½ cup	30	2	1	2 starch/bread **or** 2 fruit
Chili sauce	½ cup	30	2	1	2 starch/bread or 2 fruit
Dates	1 cup	130	4	1	8½ fruit
Raisins	½ cup	55	2	–	3½ fruit
Tomatoes or tomato juice	1 cup	9	2		2 vegetable
Tomato sauce or puree	1 cup	20	4	1	1 starch/bread **or** 4 vegetable
Sugars and Syrups:					
Corn syrup	1 cup	242	–	–	16 fruit
Gelatin, pwd. regular	3 oz. box	74	6	–	5 fruit
Honey	1 cup	264	1	–	17½ fruit
Molasses					
light	1 cup	213	–	–	14 fruit
dark	1 cup	180	–	–	12 fruit
Sugar					
brown, packed	1 cup	212	–	–	14 fruit
powdered, sifted	1 cup	100	–	–	6½ fruit
powdered, unsifted	1 cup	119	–	–	8 fruit
white	1 cup	199	–	–	13 fruit
Nuts:					
Almonds	½ cup	15	14	41	1 starch/bread 1½ med. fat meat 6½ fat
Cashews	1 cup	29	17	46	2 starch/bread 1½ med. fat meat 7½ fat

FOOD	QTY.	CARBO-HYDRATE (gm)	PROTEIN (gm)	FAT (gm)	EXCHANGES
Coconut, shredded	1 cup	33	2	24	2 fruit 5 fat
Peanuts	1 oz, ¼ cup	5	7	14	1 med. fat meat 2 fat
Peanut butter	1 cup	34	76	137	2 starch/bread 10 med. fat meat 17 fat
Pecans	1 cup	13	9	73	1 starch/bread 1 med. fat meat 13½ fat
Sunflower seed kernels	½ cup	14	17	34	1 starch/bread 2 med. fat meat 5 fat
Walnuts	1 cup	16	15	64	1 starch/bread 2 med. fat meat 10½ fat
Meats:					
Chicken, canned	5½ oz.	–	34	18	5 lean meat
Ground beef, lean	1 lb raw	–	79	66	11 med. fat meat 2 fat
Salmon, pink, canned	16 oz. can	–	93	27	13 lean meat
Tuna, water-packed	6⅛ oz. can	–	44	3	6 lean meat
Tuna, oil-packed	6½ oz. can	–	45	30	6 med. fat meat

Form 1. Converting recipes into exchanges using exchanges.

Recipe Name: _____

EXCHANGES

INGREDIENTS	STARCH	MEAT	VEGETABLES	FRUIT	MILK	FAT	FREE
Total Exchanges							
Total Exchanges ÷ Total No. of Servings							

Form 2. Example of a recipe converted into exchanges using exchange method.

Recipe Name: ___Tuna Rice Casserole (Yield: 8 servings, 1 cup)___

EXCHANGES

INGREDIENTS	STARCH	MEAT	VEGETABLES	FRUIT	MILK	FAT	FREE
1 cup wild rice	6						
¼ cup chopped onion							free
¼ cup margarine						10	
¼ cup flour	1½						
1 cup chicken broth							free
1½ cups evaporated skim milk					3		
2-6 ½ oz. cans tuna, water packed		12 lean					
¼ cup diced pimento							free
2 Tbsp. parsley							free
½ tsp. salt							free
½ tsp. pepper							free
½ cup almonds, chopped		1½ med.fat				6½	
Total Exchanges	8½	13½	0	0	3	16½	
Total Exchanges ÷ Total No. of Servings	1	2	0	0	Trace	2	

1 cup tuna rice casserole = 1 starch/bread, 2 lean meat, 2 fat exchanges **or**
1 starch/bread, 2 med. fat meat, 1 fat exchange

Form 3. Converting recipes into exchanges using grams of carbohydrate, protein, and fat.

Recipe Name: _____

NUTRIENTS

INGREDIENTS	CARBOHYDRATE GRAMS	PROTEIN GRAMS	FAT GRAMS
Total Nutrients			
Total Nutrients ÷ Total No. of Servings			

Form 4. Example of a recipe converted to exchanges using grams of carbohydrate, protein, and fat.

Recipe Name: _Sesame Cookies (Yield: 24 cookies)_

NUTRIENTS

INGREDIENTS	CARBOHYDRATE GRAMS	PROTEIN GRAMS	FAT GRAMS
2 Tbsp. sesame seeds			2
2 cups sifted flour	174	22	
¼ tsp. salt			
½ cup margarine			98
¼ cup shortening			56
1 cup sugar	199		
1 egg		6	6
1 tsp. vanilla			
Total Nutrients	**373**	**28**	**162**
Total Nutrients ÷ Total No. of Servings	16	1	7
1 starch/bread	15	3	
½ fat			8

1 cookie = 1 starch/bread, 1½ fat exchanges

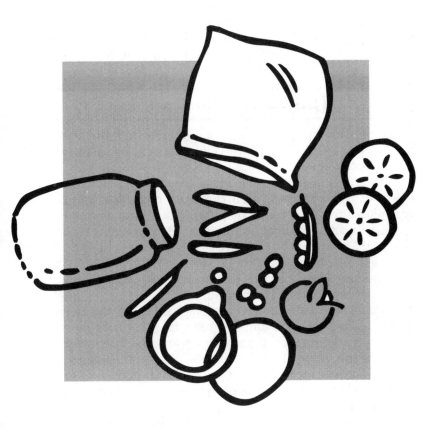

CANNING AND
FREEZING

Pride and pleasure can be yours when you preserve home-grown produce or in-season fruit market specials. Canning and freezing are easy and safe if you follow instructions carefully. Use these hints to adapt your favorite recipes for your meal plan.

Guidelines for Canning

In canning, heat is applied to a food in order to destroy microorganisms (yeasts, molds, bacteria) and to halt enzyme activity, which causes food to spoil.

The acidity of a food is one factor to consider when deciding on a method of canning. Acid occurring naturally in foods has the ability to destroy most bacteria. Therefore, a high-acid food can be preserved using a lower heat treatment, such as a boiling water bath. Low-acid foods need the pressure canning process. High-acid fruits and vegetables include apples, berries, cherries, peaches, rhubarb, and tomatoes. Low-acid vegetables include asparagus, beans, beets, carrots, corn, potatoes, and squash.

In the water bath method for high-acid fruits and vegetables, food is packed into jars and covered with a hot cooking solution. Jars are placed on a rack and quickly lowered into water. There should be two inches of water above the jars. Begin counting process time as soon as water in the canner reaches a rolling boil. Cover the canner and process with the water boiling for the recommended length of time.

Pressure canning methods should be used for low acid foods. Follow the manufacturer's directions for using pressure canners.

Packing methods include hot pack, raw or cold pack. Hot-packed food is heated thoroughly before packing. In hot packing, place fruit in a large kettle and cook until tender. Taste the cooked product and add sweetening, lemon juice, or spices as needed. The hot fruit is then packed into hot, clean jars, liquid is added to within one-half inch of the jar rim, lids are added, and the jar is boiled in the water bath. Hot-packing is good for fruits that tend to discolor and is also used for many vegetables. Raw-packing food saves time in the canning process and in some cases helps retain flavor and food value. In the raw- or cold-pack method fruit is placed directly into hot, clean jars, liquid is added to within one-half inch from the top of the jar, jar lids are screwed on, and the jar is placed into a boiling water bath or pressure cooker to process. Liquid must be added to the fruit to help the cooking process.

When cooling the jars, place them upright on dry surfaces. Let jars cool for 12 hours, then check seals. If the center of the lid holds down when pressed and the lid does not move, the jar is sealed.

Use your canned foods within one year. When opening canned food, carefully inspect the contents for signs of spoilage. Look for cloudy liquid, an "off" odor, bulging lids, deterioration, or patches of mold. Never taste doubtful food! Home canned low-acid foods should be boiled for 10 to 15 minutes before serving.

Sugar is not needed in the canning process to prevent spoilage. It is often added to fruits to help them hold shape, color, and flavor. Fruits may be easily canned without added sugar if they are canned in their own juice or water. Processing time is the same for unsweetened fruit as for sweetened. Some of the manufacturers of artificial sweeteners have guidelines for using their products in canning. Artificial sweeteners added to the canning process may produce a bitter taste. Instead you can add an artificial sweetener at serving time if you like.

Guidelines for Freezing

Fresh fruits no longer know a season. With proper freezing procedures, you can capture the beauty, texture, and taste of products from gardens and orchards.

Choose fruits that are in their prime, ripe, and firm. Prepare fruits for the way you plan to use them by peeling or slicing them. For fruits that tend to discolor, you can add lemon juice, ascorbic acid, or a compound containing ascorbic acid, such as Fruit Fresh.

Fruits are sometimes packed with sugar or syrups when frozen to add texture and flavor. This is not necessary to prevent spoilage; fruits can be packed unsweetened. (Some fruits can also be packed dry without adding liquid.) A syrup for freezing may be made from an artificial sweetener and water. The syrup should completely cover the fruit when it is used. Follow the manufacturer's directions for the amount of artificial sweetener to add to avoid a bitter taste. In addition, fruit can be artificially sweetened before serving.

Fruits and vegetables stored at 0° F or below will maintain high quality for 8 to 12 months. However, unsweetened fruit tends to lose quality more rapidly, so include these foods in your menus as soon as feasible.

Tips on Preserving Without Sugar

For canning fruits, use the water bath method and artificially sweetened syrup. Then process the fruit the same as fruit canned in sugar syrup. Pack peaches, pears, and apricots raw in pint jars; add boiling water or syrup to cover the fruit; wipe off the jar rim; place a lid and ring on firmly; and process the jar for 25 minutes in a boiling water bath. For pears and peaches, add one teaspoon of an ascorbic-acid-type fruit freshener (such as Fruit Fresh) per pint of syrup to keep the fruit from darkening.

Prepare plums and cherries in the same way. Prick them instead of removing the pits. The process time is 20 minutes for pint jars. Plums, if fully ripe when canned, are fine in a water pack. The other fruits seem more flavorful when canned in an artificially sweetened syrup. Make the syrup with one tablespoon liquid sweetener for each pint of boiling water. Pour the syrup into the jars while it is boiling hot.

Put hot unsweetened applesauce into pint jars and process for 25 minutes in a boiling water bath. The sweetness of applesauce depends on the variety and ripeness of the apple. Sweetener can be added to applesauce just before serving. Check the jars when they are cool to make sure the lids are sealed. Store them in a cool place.

Fruits can also be canned without sugar using a syrup made from fruit juice. When using the canned fruit with the juice, be sure to count the carbohydrate in the juice as well as in the fruit. One-half cup fruit equals one fruit exchange; one half-cup fruit with one third cup of juice equals two fruit exchanges.

To make the fruit juice syrup use:
⅓ cup orange juice
4 cups liquified fruit
(peach, pear, etc. pureed in blender)
1½ cups white grape juice (Catawba)

7¾ cups water

Cook for five minutes at boiling and then reduce heat. Pour it over fruit and process canned fruit in a boiling water bath for 30 minutes.

Or make the following syrup and follow the same procedure.

10 cups water

⅓ cup orange juice

1½ cups white grape juice (Catawba)

Raspberries, strawberries, and cantaloupe balls or chunks can be frozen without sugar or syrup. Use small containers that hold no more than a cup. There is some vitamin loss in freezing them "dry," but it is well worth the loss to have the color and flavor of these fruits available during the winter months.

Guidelines for Sugar-Free Jams and Jellies

Tasty sugarless or lower sugar jams and jellies can be made from fruit. Grape or apple jellies can be made using unsweetened, either canned or frozen, juices. In a saucepan, soften 2 packages or 2 tablespoons unflavored gelatin in 1 quart apple juice or 1 bottle (24 ounces) grape juice and 2 tablespoons lemon juice. Bring to a rolling boil, dissolving gelatin; boil 1 minute. Remove from heat. Stir in 2 tablespoons liquid artificial sweetener and food coloring, if desired. Pour hot into jars. Adjust caps. Store in refrigerator up to three weeks. Yield: about 1 to 2 pints. One tablespoon = 8 to 11 calories.

Sugarless peach, raspberry, or strawberry jam can also be made and frozen. Crush 1 quart of any of the fruits in a saucepan. Stir in 3 to 4 teaspoons liquid artificial sweetener, 2 teaspoons lemon juice, and 1 package powdered pectin (and for peaches, ½ teaspoon ascorbic acid). Bring to a boil; boil 1 minute. Remove from heat. Continue to stir 2 minutes. Pour into freeze jars. Adjust caps. Freeze. Yield: about 1 pint. One tablespoon = 5 to 8 calories.

You can also make homemade jams and jellies using Light Sure-Jell, which is fruit pectin. You will use about half the sugar that is used for making jams and jellies using Sure-Jell. Do not reduce the amount of sugar called for in the recipe or use a sugar substitute. The exact amounts listed in the recipe of sugar, fruit, and pectin are necessary for a good set. Follow the directions that come with

Light Sure-Jell and it will result in jams and jellies with about half the calories of regular jams and jellies. Two teaspoons = 14 to 16 calories.

Do not substitute artificial sweetener for sugar in a regular jam or jelly recipe. It will be oversweet and taste very bitter. When making jam with light colored fruits, add two teaspoons of Fruit Fresh to retain the bright color.

And finally—enjoy!

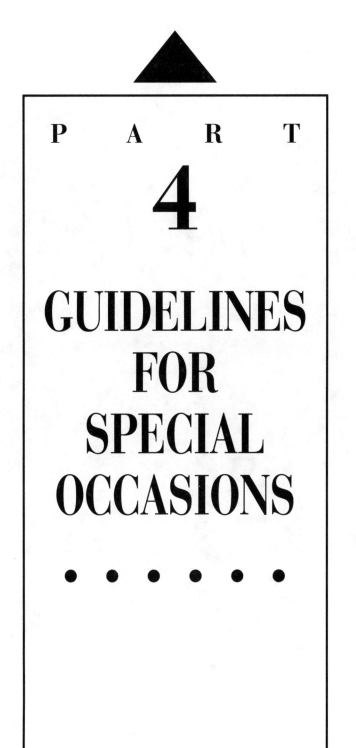

P A R T

4

GUIDELINES
FOR
SPECIAL
OCCASIONS

• • • • • •

30

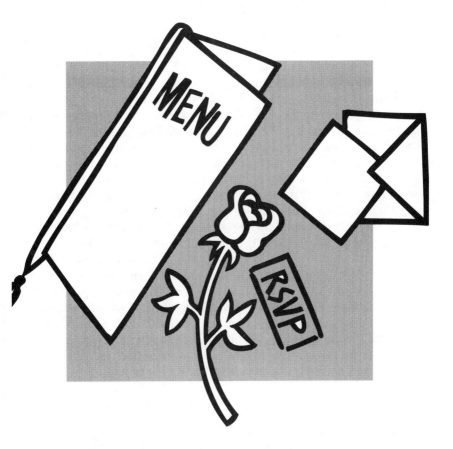

UNDERSTAND YOUR MEAL PLAN AND ENJOY DINING OUT

When Americans dine out—and they are doing this more than ever—reports indicate they aren't leaving their taste for a healthy diet at home. In 1989, 39 percent of consumers surveyed reported they chose what they consider nutritious items when dining out compared to 35 percent in 1986. But calorie for calorie, foods eaten away from home have more fat and lower levels of nutrients than foods eaten at home. So be choosy!

Dining out is on the rise. A survey of consumers and restaurant managers conducted in 1990 by the National Restaurant Association showed that 42 percent of the food dollar was spent away from home, in comparison with 24 percent in 1950. On the average Americans eat more than a third of meals away from home—about one a day. The art of menu reading is no longer a luxury but a necessity. Are you part of this large group of consumers eating meals out in restaurants or one of the increasing number of individuals purchasing meals at restaurants or delicatessens to eat at home?

A growing number of restaurants and delicatessens are actively promoting nutrition or low-calorie fare. Almost three out of four restaurants report they will alter the way they prepare foods at a diner's request. Almost all restaurants will serve a sauce or salad dressing on the side or cook without salt. Most will cook with margarine or vegetable oil and help diners who are trying to limit their intake of saturated fats. Four out of five restaurants will broil or bake a food instead of frying it. There are more choices available today.

Sauces and cooking techniques can make the difference between low-fat cuisine and high-calorie, high-fat meals. Chicken, turkey, fish, or lean red meat can be the start of a healthy dish, but adding mayonnaise-based dressings, butter, or cream-based sauces, and cooking techniques using oil turn the final product into a high-fat choice.

How often you eat out also determines how careful you need to be in the selection of menu choices. If you eat more than five meals per week out, then your meals need to closely match your meal plan. If you rarely eat out—once a month or to celebrate a special occasion—you can take more liberties with your selections.

When eating at a restaurant, cafeteria, or friend's home or when purchasing food from a delicatessen, bring your good common sense with you. You can follow your meal plan and enjoy yourself at the same time. Knowledge of food values should enable anyone to select proper items from fairly varied menus. For gastronomical adventures, follow these simple guidelines.

Guidelines

Know your meal plan. Know how many exchanges you are allowed for each meal and then make selections accordingly. Most menus include appetizers, soups, entrees, breads, salads, and desserts. You can generally determine which food group a selection on the menu falls into. Use your exchanges wisely.

Carrying a wallet-sized summary of your meal plan, which lists the exchanges or number of servings for the foods you routinely eat, can be a helpful reminder.

Watch portion sizes. Be familiar with your usual portion size so you will be able to judge correctly what you should eat. Don't feel you have to eat all the food served. If portion sizes are too large for your meal plan, share your entree, leave the food, or ask for a "doggie bag." You can save that extra food for lunch the next day. If you have diabetes, remember it's more important to keep your diabetes under control than to clean your plate!

Train your eyes to measure portion sizes. You can develop this ability at home by using measuring utensils to get the right portions of familiar foods. When you become a good eyeball judge, occasionally check your accuracy. It's easy for teaspoons of margarine, tablespoons of salad dressings, or half-cups of mashed potatoes to become larger and larger!

Learn how to estimate the exchanges and calories for unfamiliar foods. If the food is meat, fish, or poultry, then regardless of its exotic name, a one-ounce serving will equal one meat exchange. If it is a starch, a half-cup serving of pastas or starchy vegetables or one ounce of a bread product (about the weight and size of a medium-sized dinner roll) will equal one starch/bread exchange and about 15 grams of carbohydrate. The equivalent of a small- to medium-sized fresh fruit will be one fruit exchange.

Take charge—ask questions. If you are not sure how a dish is prepared, ask the person waiting on you. You should ask not only about how a certain item is prepared, but also about the portion size. Find out how many ounces of meat, fish, potatoes, or vegetables are in a standard portion. Most restaurants use standard portion sizes since this allows them to properly price the item on their menus.

Be assertive in requesting how you want your meal served—you are the one paying for it! For example, you can ask that your food not be buttered before broiling, that a sauce be omitted or served on the side so you can control the amount, or that a high-fat cheese to be melted on top be omitted.

Watch preparation. Consider how the food was prepared—was it broiled, baked, roasted, fried, or breaded? What accompanies the selection—gravy, whipping cream, sour cream? While you are still learning, it may be wise to select simply prepared foods and avoid rich sauces and casseroles with many ingredients.

How foods are cooked affects their exchange value. Meat weight listed on a menu refers to the portion size before cooking. Meat loses about a fourth of its weight in cooking, so an eight-ounce steak is approximately six, not eight, meat exchanges after it is cooked. Additionally, foods breaded and fried in deep fat, such as chicken and shrimp, contain an additional starch/bread exchange and one to two additional fat exchanges per serving.

Choose foods described as broiled (ask about added butter), roasted, steamed, poached, or stir-fried. Foods with tomato or cocktail sauces, or in broth or wine, are nutrition winners. Avoid foods described as buttery, sauteed, pan- or deep-fried, creamed, escalloped, or au gratin. Watch out for cream, butter, cheese, and hollandaise sauces as well.

Request that condiments, such as salad dressings, gravy, sauces, and so on, be served separately. By having them served on the side, you can control the amounts. That way you can eat only small quantities of fats such as salad dressings, butter or margarine, gravies, sauces, whipped cream, and sour cream.

Use low- or reduced-calorie and diet products when available. Some restaurants now have diet syrups, jams, and jellies and low- or reduced-calorie salad dressings. These items may not appear on the menu but may be available if you ask for them.

Plan ahead. You can move one meat exchange and all the fat exchanges you can spare from another time of day to your meal out. It is a good idea to save as many fat exchanges as you can, because meals out usually contain more fat than meals at home. (You might even try to be careful of fat exchanges the next day as well!)

Know which food groups can be exchanged for other food groups. The easiest interchange is between the fruit and starch/bread lists:

1 fruit = 1 starch/bread and/or 1 starch/bread = 1 fruit exchange

If fruit is not available, you can have another starch/bread serving instead. This is helpful because often the starch servings are larger in restaurants than what you have at home. Or you would like to have a piece of garlic toast. If you wish more fruit than is allowed on your meal plan, use a starch/bread exchange. A fresh fruit plate may be a good choice for lunch but you may need to use all of your starch/bread exchanges as fruit exchanges.

1 nonfat milk = 1 starch/bread plus 1 lean meat (It really should be one nonfat milk and 1 fat exchange; however, when you eat out you'll probably find that you're short of fat exchanges.) This is a helpful interchange when you would prefer a larger serving of meat and starch instead of milk.

Adjust meal and insulin injection times. Persons taking insulin must remember to eat on schedule. But sometimes it is necessary to delay meals because of social commitments or work. If a meal is delayed by one hour, have a fruit or starch/bread exchange (15 grams of carbohydrate) at the scheduled meal time. This is particularly important if you take your insulin injection at the usual time.

If your meal is delayed for longer than 1½ hours, you have several options. The first option is to move the evening snack to the mealtime and have the meal later. (This option is especially important if you are taking only one injection of insulin in the morning.)

If you take two injections of insulin, another option may be better. If dinner is not delayed more than 1½ hours, you can wait and take your insulin before the meal and then have your snack at the usual time. Delaying the second injection too long, however, may cause an overlap of intermediate-acting insulin the next morning. To prevent this you can use the third option. Take your dinner intermediate-acting insulin at the usual time and take the regular before your meal. When you take your intermediate-acting insulin, eat half of your evening snack. When you have dinner, eat the rest of your snack. Check your blood glucose before going to bed to see if an additional snack is needed.

Of course, if you take an intermediate-acting insulin before bed you can continue to do that and simply have the regular insulin before dinner. If dinner is delayed too long it may be a good idea to have a fruit or a starch/bread exchange from your evening snack at your usual dinnertime.

If brunch is the meal you are planning to eat out, follow your usual morning routine and eat a small breakfast (1–2 starch/breads), have brunch in place of your morning snack (remaining breakfast exchanges plus lunch exchanges), and eat your morning snack at your usual lunchtime.

Making any of these changes will probably affect your blood glucose readings because you may be testing closer to your large meal than you normally do.

Oops! If you feel you have indeed "blown it," remember that you can exercise! Granted, it takes a lot of exercise to burn many calories, but dancing, bicycling, or walking briskly can help.

An important word of caution: If you find your bedtime blood glucose level is higher than usual, do NOT take extra regular insulin at that time. If you thought you would do okay and then find you "blew it," taking extra regular insulin after the fact really won't help much. By the time the insulin is at its peak of action the elevated blood glucose from the meal will have decreased. The time to take extra regular insulin is *before* a meal—not after. Also, it should only be one or two extra units—not five or ten as many individuals want to add. Check with your health care team on how to make adjustments in your insulin before your meal.

Understand restaurant menu terms. This can help you find low-fat preparations and avoid high-fat dishes on menus. The following guide to restaurant terms can help you recognize preparation methods. A la Grecque, au maigre, cacciatore, chasseur, creole, deviled, jambalaya (without sausage), julienne, marinara, and scallopine, if prepared with low-fat ingredients, are good choices and can add spice, variety, and interest to meals without adding excessive amounts of fat and calories.

Menu Item   Preparation and Ingredients

A la Grecque Usually cooked in oil and vinegar or lemon juice with seasonings.

A la King A white sauce with mushrooms and pimiento or green pepper.

Au Gratin Cooking process that produces a crisp, golden brown crust, usually formed by baking or broiling bread crumbs, cheese, and butter; or dishes that will crust on their own accord.

Au Jus Meat served in its own juice.

Au Maigre With no meat.

Bearnaise Rich sauce made with egg yolks, tarragon, butter, shallots, vinegar, and sometimes white wine.

Bordelaise Brown sauce seasoned with wine and shallots, garnished with poached marrow and parsley.

Cacciatore Tomato sauce with mushrooms, herbs, and other seasonings.

Chasseur (Hunter's Sauce) Brown sauce with tomatoes, mushrooms, herbs, and other seasonings.

Coq au Vin Sauteed in red wine and brown sauce with mushrooms and onions.

Creole Spicy combination of tomatoes, green peppers, okra, onions, and seasonings, usually cooked in oil.

Deviled Prepared with hot or savory seasoning usually after being finely chopped.

Hollandaise Usually made with egg yolks, butter, lemon juice, or vinegar.

Jambalaya Spicy dish of rice, tomatoes, onions, peppers, and other seasonings; usually includes sausage.

Julienne Cut into matchlike strips.

Kiev Stuffed with seasoned butter and flour; often deep-fried in oil.

Kippered Lightly salted and smoked.

Lyonnaise	Cooked with pieces of onion and butter.
Marinara	Tomato-based sauce with onion, garlic, and seasonings.
Mornay	A bechamel sauce with cream and grated cheese, sometimes egg yolks.
Parmigiana	Covered with bread crumbs and Parmesan cheese, then sauteed in butter and served with tomato sauce; usually includes mozzarella cheese as well.
Remoulade	Chopped pickles and capers with mayonnaise, tarragon, and spices.
Scallopine	Meat pounded very thin, floured, and broiled or sauteed in wine sauce.
Thermidor	Cream sauce seasoned with wine and herbs or mustard.

In summary, when dining away from home, it's helpful to do some planning. Plan where you will eat, what you will eat, and how much you will eat.

▲ **Where:** It helps if you're familiar with the menu of the restaurant. The more choices on the menu, the more apt you are to find choices appropriate for you.

▲ **What:** Of primary importance is familiarity with your meal plan. Decide ahead of time what you are going to order that fits into your meal plan. By doing this you won't be tempted by inappropriate food choices. Be the trendsetter—order first. Have you noticed how often the rest of the table orders what the first person chooses? By ordering first you won't be as apt to be influenced by what the others order and better yet, they will probably follow your example—and all will benefit!

▲ **How Much:** Judging portion sizes by "eyeballing" them will help you decide how much to take home and save for another meal.

By planning, understanding your meal plan, and correctly judging portion sizes, you can enjoy dining away from home while keeping your weight and/or your diabetes in control.

Good Choices

Appetizers: Tomato juice and other vegetable juices, fruit juice, broth-or tomato-based soup, bouillon, consommé, raw vegetable platter, fresh fruit cocktail, shrimp or crab cocktail with cocktail sauce.

Entrees: Roasted, baked, broiled, blackened, grilled, stir-fried, or barbecued meat, fish, poultry, or seafood.

Ask that gravy or sauces be served on the side. Some restaurants will add fats to meat or fish before broiling. If the serving exceeds your portion size (bigger than a deck of cards), either share it with a companion or remember the doggie bag. Instead of a large entree, order an appetizer portion.

Filet mignon or shish kebobs are good choices when ordering beef; the portion size is reasonable and the meat is lean. Broiled quarter-pounders without the high-fat sauces are about 3 meat exchanges.

Steamed clams or softshell crab; broiled or steamed lobster (be careful of butter); grilled scallops; steamed crab or crab claws; mussels; venison; leg of lamb, fat trimmed; teriyaki-style chicken or beef; chicken or beef fajitas.

Chili; turkey club sandwich (hold the mayonnaise); roast beef or ham sandwich (mustard only); grilled chicken sandwiches; pita sandwiches; pasta with vegetables and tomato-based sauce; vegetable, barley, meat, poultry, or fish-based soups; lentil, black bean, or split pea soups.

Starches: Mashed, baked, broiled, or steamed potatoes; steamed rice or rice pilaf; noodles; corn on the cob.

Ask for the butter, margarine, or sour cream to be on the side so you can govern the portion used.

Breads: Order breads that are not frosted or glazed.

For variety, substitute hard or soft dinner rolls; French bread (3" slice); pita bread, rye, pumpernickel, or sourdough breads or rolls; plain muffin; crackers; popovers.

| | Other substitutes for one starch/bread exchange: two 8" long bread sticks, 4 melba toast rectangles or 8 rounds, 4 Ry-Krisp, ½ bagel or English muffin, ½ hamburger or hot dog bun (one if small or about 1 oz.). |

Salads: Vegetable or fresh fruit salads.

Use a lemon wedge, vinegar, or known amount of dressing. (One tablespoon of regular dressing equals 1 fat exchange; 2 to 3 tablespoons of a low- or reduced-calorie dressing equals 1 fat exchange.)

At salad bars, fill your plate with raw vegetables (count a large plate filled from the salad bar as 3 vegetables or 1 starch/bread [15 grams of carbohydrate]) and top sparingly with high-calorie items—cheese, olives, seeds, croutons, hard-boiled eggs, and bacon. Skip the salads made with mayonnaise-based dressings—potato, pasta, coleslaw, and so on.

Vegetables: Raw, stewed, steamed, boiled, broiled, stir-fried, or baked. Allow for a fat serving if vegetables are flavored with butter, margarine, or oil.

Avoid vegetables with a glaze or sweet and sour sauce, or that are deep-fried. Ask for a baked potato plain or with margarine or sour cream served separately. Remember that peas, corn, lima beans, and winter squash are considered starch/breads.

Fruit: Fresh fruit, fresh fruit salad, or fruit juices.

Desserts: Fresh fruit, frozen nonfat yogurt, plain ice cream or sherbet, fresh fruit sorbet, sponge cake, or angel food cake.

Fats: Margarine, butter, salad dressing, sour cream. Be careful of amounts. Instead of mayonnaise or butter on sandwiches, use mustard, horseradish, pickles, and/or lettuce, tomatoes.

Beverages: Coffee, tea, skim milk, diet soft drinks, mineral water.

For other suggestions see Section II, Chapters 14 to 17, for ethnic choices; Chapter 19 for fast-food selections.

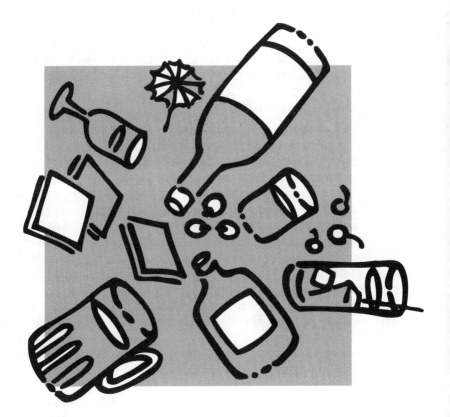

IF ALCOHOL IS USED

For many persons alcoholic beverages have become an accepted part of their social lives. The decision to drink or not drink alcoholic beverages must be made by each individual. To make this decision, you need to be aware of the effects of alcohol on the body, and if you have diabetes, the effect of alcohol on blood glucose control.

Metabolism of Alcohol

Research has shown how the body deals with alcohol and why it is damaging, particularly to the liver and brain, if taken in excess.

Alcohol is broken down in the liver by specific enzymes, but the liver can process less than one ounce of alcohol in an hour. When more than that amount enters the liver, it moves through the liver into the general blood circulation. When this happens, alcohol reaches the central nervous system and eventually the brain and the effects of alcohol on behavior begin. Initially it lifts the barriers of self-control, but alcohol is a depressant and it will eventually slow down brain activity. When the liver can handle the alcohol it will be recirculated to the liver and metabolized.

Alcohol cannot be converted to glucose by the liver, but it can be used as a source of energy. If the calories from alcohol are not used as an immediate energy source, they are converted to fat and triglycerides. (This is why if individuals drink too much alcohol they develop a fatty liver. It is also why alcohol can be the cause of high blood triglyceride levels.)

The metabolism of alcohol does not require insulin. In fact, alcohol increases the effect of insulin. Alcohol does not stimulate the pancreas to release insulin, but it enhances the glucose-lowering action of insulin or other hypoglycemic agents. The presence of alcohol has also been shown to prolong the effects of a single injection of insulin.

Overall, alcohol lowers blood glucose levels, especially if it has been some time since food was eaten. In that case, blood glucose is initially supplied by the breakdown of carbohydrate stored in the liver (glycogen) and later by the liver's conversion of protein to glucose. Alcohol inhibits this conversion of protein to glucose, which causes hypoglycemia (too low a blood glucose level). Furthermore, release of "stress hormones" that raise blood glucose levels becomes blunted, increasing the risk for hypoglycemic reactions becoming more severe.

Hypoglycemia can occur even before a person is aware of being mildly intoxicated. If food has not been eaten for several hours before or with the alcoholic beverage, two ounces of alcohol is enough to produce hypoglycemia. Also, persons in poor control of their diabetes or who have exercised strenuously usually have depleted carbohydrate stores and so are at special risk for hypoglycemia.

Even when alcohol is consumed with food, the hypoglycemic action of alcohol may persist from 8 to 12 hours after the last drink and may occur after only one drink or two. At this point, the body needs to convert protein to blood glucose but alcohol blocks the process.

On occasion, alcohol can cause blood glucose levels to become elevated. This may be because alcohol affects judgment, making it difficult for a person to follow a meal plan. However, this hyperglycemia is usually temporary and is followed several hours later by a drop in blood glucose to below-normal levels.

Alcohol is a concentrated source of calories, yielding seven calories per gram. For comparison, carbohydrate and protein contribute four calories per gram and fat contributes nine calories per gram. Alcohol provides energy but no other essential nutrients. An ounce and a half of 80 proof liquor contributes 100 calories. Sweet wines and beers also contain carbohydrates, so they have additional calories.

When diabetes is well controlled, the blood glucose level is not affected by the moderate use of alcohol if it is consumed shortly before, during, or immediately after eating. However, alcohol should be avoided in certain conditions: alcohol abuse, elevated triglyceride levels, gastritis, pancreatitis, certain types of kidney and heart diseases, frequent hypoglycemic reactions, gestational diabetes, type I diabetes with pregnancy. Check with your health care team to determine whether any of these contraindications applies to you. Alcohol also interacts with barbiturates and tranquilizers, sleeping pills, antihistamines, cold remedies, and a number of drugs. Avoid these combinations.

Guidelines for the Use of Alcohol

Many persons with diabetes can include alcohol with their meal plan by following some simple guidelines. These guidelines refer to occasional use of alcoholic beverages, which is defined as about two "equivalents" (drinks) not more than once or twice a week. If alcohol is used daily, the amount must be limited and the calories counted in the meal plan.

The guidelines listed below can help persons with diabetes make informed decisions about the use of alcohol.

▲ **Drink alcohol only if your diabetes is in good control.** Drinking alcohol when you are in poor control can make control even worse. Your health care team can advise you on how to balance your food intake, exercise, and medication to achieve better blood glucose control, and they will tell you if there is some reason you should avoid alcoholic beverages. To keep control of your diabetes, know the effect of alcohol on blood glucose levels.

▲ **Drink alcohol in moderation.** Sip slowly and make a drink last a long time. Even one drink is enough to give the breath the smell of alcohol. Since symptoms of alcohol intoxication and hypoglycemia are similar, it is easy for other people to mistake the low blood sugar for intoxication and delay necessary treatment.

▲ **Limit yourself to no more than two of the following equivalents, or drinks, each day.** Each contains about the same amount of alcohol.

  – 1.5 oz of distilled spirits (hard liquor such as whiskey, scotch, rye, vodka, gin, cognac, rum, dry brandy)
  – 4 oz of dry wine
  – 2 oz of dry sherry
  – 12 oz of beer, preferably light

▲ **For persons of normal weight who take injected insulin, two of the above drinks can occasionally be used as an "extra."** No food should be omitted because of the possibility of alcohol-induced hypoglycemia and because alcohol does not require insulin to be metabolized. However, even this amount of alcohol can cause hypoglycemia if not accompanied by food.

▲ **Persons with Type II diabetes for whom weight is a concern must count the calories from alcohol in their meal plan.** Calories are best substituted for fat exchanges because alcohol is metabolized in a manner similar to fat (each of the above equivalents is equal to two fat exchanges). Avoid or limit alcohol consumption if you need to shed excess pounds. Since alcohol provides calories (without the benefit of other nutrients), most of which your body stores as fat, losing weight may become more difficult when you drink, even occasionally.

▲ **Never drink on an empty stomach or after vigorous exercise.** Alcohol (as does exercise) makes you especially vulnerable to hypoglycemia, so be sure to drink only with, directly before, or shortly after a meal. Remember that alcohol may also promote hypoglycemia the "morning after."

▲ **Avoid drinks that contain large amounts of carbohydrate.** Liqueurs and cordials are sweet and may have a sugar content as high as 50 percent. Beer and ale contain malt sugar, which should be substituted in the meal plan. Light beer is recommended because it has about 3 to 6 grams of carbohydrate in a 12-ounce can, in contrast to regular beer, which has 13 grams of carbohydrate per can.

▲ **Don't let a drink make you careless.** Alcohol can have a relaxing effect and may dull judgment. Be sure meals and snacks are taken on time and selected with usual care. Too much alcohol may lead to further dietary indiscretion. Avoid hypoglycemia the morning after drinking alcohol by setting your alarm before you retire to help you get up, test your blood glucose, and eat your usual breakfast.

▲ **Carry identification.** Visible identification should be carried or worn when drinking away from home. An insulin reaction can appear too much like intoxication to take any chances.

Composition of Alcoholic Beverages

▲ **Beer** is made by fermenting grain mash (barley grains) to malt sugar, which is partially converted to ethanol (alcohol). Beers

vary in alcohol content from 3.2 percent to 4.5 percent for
light-colored beers to 6 percent to 7 percent for darker beers.
A typical 12-ounce serving of regular beer contains 13 to 18
grams of carbohydrate and has 150 calories.

▲ **Light beers** have considerably less carbohydrate and slightly
less alcohol than regular beer. They contain 3 to 6 grams of
carbohydrate in a 12-ounce serving and 90 to 100 calories.

▲ **Near beer** is brewed in the same manner as regular beer, but
an additional process produces a near nonalcoholic malt beverage. A 12-ounce serving contains about 12 grams of carbohydrate and 60 calories.

▲ **Distilled spirits** are grain mash, sugar cane, molasses, or fruit
juices fermented to ethanol. By distilling the fermented products a higher concentration of alcohol in distilled spirits is
achieved. Proof is the measure of alcohol content. The percentage of alcohol content is found by dividing the proof in
half. For example, 80-proof whiskey is 40 percent alcohol.
Distilled spirits have a high alcohol content with virtually no
carbohydrate. One and one-half ounces of 80-proof distilled
spirits contain 14 grams of alcohol and 100 calories.

▲ **Wines** are made by fermenting the juice of grapes, berries or
other fruits, dandelions, honey, or rice. They are dry or sweet
depending on whether or not all the sugar has been allowed to
change to alcohol. The alcohol content varies from 9 percent
to 20 percent, with an average of 11.5 percent. The higher
percentages occur in sherry, port, and sake. An average serving of 4 ounces of a **dry wine** contains 12 grams of alcohol and
.1 percent to .3 percent carbohydrate; **sweet wines** have a
higher sugar content, and sweet kosher wines can approach
15 percent or more carbohydrate.

Wines with a low carbohydrate content (less than 2 percent
sugar) include red wines (burgundy, cabernet, sauvignon,
claret, gamay beaujolais, and merlot), white wines (chablis,
chardonnay, dry chenin blanc, French colombard, dry ries-
lings, dry sauterne, dry sauvignon blanc, white burgundy), and
other wines such as dry rose, dry champagne, and dry sherry.

▲ **Wine coolers** are combinations of wine and fruit juice, usually in equal portions, to which carbonation and a sweetener have been added. A typical 12-ounce serving of a wine cooler contains 30 grams of carbohydrate (120 calories) and 13 grams of alcohol (90 calories) for a total of 210 calories.

▲ **De-alcoholized wines** are basically fruit juice; 4 ounces contain 7 grams of carbohydrate and 35 calories.

▲ **Liqueurs (or cordials)** are sweet with a sugar content as high as 50 percent and alcohol content from 20 percent to 55 percent. One cordial glass (⅔ ounce) contains 6 to 7 grams of carbohydrate and 6 to 7 grams of alcohol, with about 65 to 75 calories.

▲ **Sherries** that are dry are low in carbohydrate (less than 2 grams per 2-ounce serving), whereas **sweet sherries, port, and muscatel (dessert wine)** contain 7 grams of carbohydrate per 2-ounce serving.

▲ **Cocktails** average 33 percent alcohol and contribute 110 to 180 calories per serving.

The following table on alcoholic beverages provides information on the average alcohol, carbohydrate, and calorie content of alcoholic beverages and exchanges for persons concerned about weight.

▲ ALCOHOLIC BEVERAGES ▲

BEVERAGE	SERVING	ALCO-HOL (gms)	CARBO-HYDRATE (gms)	CAL-ORIES	EXCHANGES for Type II
Beer					
regular	12 oz	13	13	150	1 starch, 2 fat
light	12 oz	11	5	100	2 fat
near	12 oz	1.5	12	60	1 starch
Distilled Spirits					
80 proof (gin, rum, vodka, whiskey, scotch)	1½ oz	14	trace	100	2 fat
dry brandy, cognac	1 oz	11	trace	75	1½ fat

BEVERAGE	SERVING	ALCO-HOL (gms)	CARBO-HYDRATE (gms)	CAL-ORIES	EXCHANGES for Type II
Table Wines					
dry white	4 oz	11	trace	80	2 fat
red or rosé	4 oz	12	trace	85	2 fat
sweet	4 oz	12	5	105	⅓ starch, 2 fat
light	4 oz	6	1	50	1 fat
wine cooler	4 oz	13	30	215	2 fruit, 2 fat
Sparkling Wines					
champagne	4 oz	12	4	100	2 fat
sweet kosher	4 oz	12	12	132	1 starch, 2 fat
Appetizer/Dessert Wines					
sherry	2 oz	9	2	74	1½ fat
sweet sherry, port, muscatel	2 oz	9	7	90	½ starch, 1½ fat
cordials, liqueurs	1½ oz	13	18	160	1 starch, 2 fat
Cocktails					
Bloody Mary	5 oz	14	5	116	1 vegetable, 2 fat
Daiquiri	2 oz	14	2	111	2 fat
Manhattan	2 oz	17	2	178	2½ fat
Martini	2½ oz	22	trace	156	3½ fat
Old-Fashioned	4 oz	26	trace	180	4 fat
Tom Collins	7½ oz	16	3	120	2½ fat
Mixes					
mineral water	any	–	0	0	Free
sugar-free tonic	any	–	0	0	Free
club soda	any	–	0	0	Free
diet soda	any	–	0	0	Free
tomato juice	½ cup	–	5	25	1 vegetable
Bloody Mary mix	½ cup	–	5	25	1 vegetable
orange juice	½ cup	–	15	60	1 fruit
grapefruit juice	½ cup	–	15	60	1 fruit
pineapple juice	½ cup	–	15	60	1 fruit

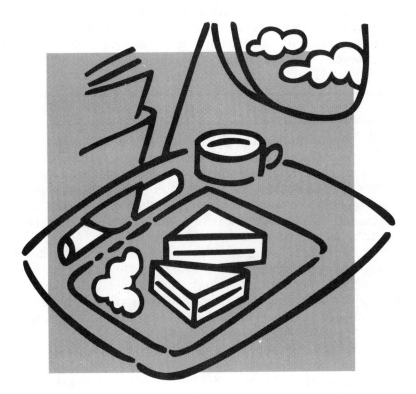

MAKE MEAL PLANNING PART OF TRAVEL PLANNING

Planning is essential before taking any trip—a one day excursion, a weekend camping trip, or international travel. Taking appropriate precautions and planning your trip with your diabetes in mind make travel safer and more enjoyable. The following tips are offered to assist you in your planning.

Guidelines

Keep your diabetes in good control. You will want to avoid insulin reactions and chances of ketoacidosis so you can fully enjoy your time away. To do this you must regularly monitor your blood glucose and follow your meal plan. Unfortunately, some people feel they would like to take a vacation from their diabetes when they are away from home. This can cause serious problems.

Take all necessary diabetes-related supplies. Always carry insulin, syringes, blood glucose monitoring equipment, and urine ketone testing materials with you. Bring extra Regular insulin along to use if you become ill. You don't want to spend precious travel time trying to find glucose strips, insulin, or syringes. Pack these necessities in a carry-on bag instead of a checked through suitcase to avoid major problems if the suitcase is lost.

If you plan to be gone for a long time, you may want to contact your insulin manufacturer to make sure insulin is available in the country you will be visiting. A foreign country may carry the insulin you use, but it may have a different name. U-100 insulin and U-100 syringes are not available in all countries.

Protect your strips and insulin from extremes in temperature—temperatures above 86 degrees or below freezing may produce inaccurate results. You can keep your insulin in a plastic bag in a wide-mouthed thermos jug lined with a wet washcloth. This way, the insulin stays cool and the vials won't break.

A well-equipped medical kit containing bandages, antiseptic solution, a decongestant, motion sickness pills, and sunscreen is also invaluable to the traveler.

Carry identification. Always carry a card in your wallet and wear a wristband or necklace bearing medical identification.

Charms and bracelets are available from the Medic Alert Foundation, International (P.O. Box 1009, Turlock, CA 95381-10009. Telephone: 800-344-3226). Travel companions should be aware that you have diabetes and should know what to do in case of an emergency such as hypoglycemia or hyperglycemia.

Schedules. Schedules, whether you travel by airplane, bus, or train, are frequently changed. Delays are often encountered. Always carry extra food for these emergencies. Another well-planned kit with supplies for diabetes-related emergencies can prevent significant problems when traveling.

Changing time zones. If you plan to jet across several time zones, you need advice on how to adjust your insulin. There are some general guidelines for adjusting your insulin when crossing time zones. When you lose hours from your day, such as what happens when traveling east from the United States to Europe, you may need a schedule of Regular insulin only and/or a reduction in your intermediate-acting insulin, NPH or Lente. One method that can be used is to decrease the intermediate-acting insulin by whatever percentage of the day you are going to be losing. For example, if the time difference is 6 hours (24 divided by 6), you would decrease NPH or Lente by 25 percent.

When adding hours to your day, such as when traveling west from Europe to the United States, you may need an extra dose of Regular insulin. Another method is to use the premeal Regular insulin as a supplement. Before meals you increase your Regular insulin by 10 percent of your usual 24-hour dose. For example, if in a day the total amount of Regular and NPH or Lente insulin you take is 40 units, you would increase your usual Regular insulin by 4 units before meals. It is very important that you consult your health care team well in advance of travel for an individualized food and insulin schedule. As you can see, different methods can be used to adjust insulin to accommodate time changes.

A group in Helsinki, Finland, reported on a study they conducted in which they advised persons with diabetes on how to adjust their insulin regime during long-distance flights. When traveling east, they caught flights that left between 5 p.m. and 9 p.m. After departure they took their normal or a slightly reduced dose of dinnertime or bedtime intermediate-acting insulin. In addition, they took an extra dose of 2 to 6 units of Regular insulin before the late meal on the plane. The next morning the usual dose of Regular insulin was taken according to local time but reduced by 20 to 40 percent because it was taken later than usual.

When traveling west, they used their normal insulin regimen until departure and then followed it according to the local time after landing. The additional hours due to the shift in time zones were covered with one or two injections of Regular insulin with meals on the plane. The additional Regular dose was about 20 to 30 percent of the total dose.

All were advised to test their blood glucose frequently. As a result of these changes the average blood glucose was only 27 mg/dl higher during westward travel and 40 mg/dl higher during eastward travel than that during days at home. They concluded that careful planning of an insulin regimen, together with monitoring of blood glucose levels, maintains good glucose control and increases safety for persons with diabetes during travel.

When traveling in the United States and the time change is only one, two, or three hours you can gradually change your morning insulin injection time. Each morning move it one-half hour ahead or behind—depending on which direction you are going—until you are back on schedule.

Flying and meals. When you book your flight, you can order a special meal through your travel agent or the airline. You must make your request at least forty-eight hours ahead of departure. They can plan for a diabetic meal to be served to you as part of the in-flight service. Sometimes the low-cholesterol meal is more appropriate than the diabetic meal, or consider the fresh fruit plate, steamed vegetable platter, or seafood salad that most airlines offer. When boarding the plane, tell the flight attendant that you have diabetes, that you have ordered a special meal, and that it is important to have your meals served on time.

Have some nonperishable foods with you in your pocket, purse, or flight bag — a box of raisins, dried fruit, or small can of fruit juice are easy to carry.

Sometimes the special meal doesn't arrive, even if you have ordered it well in advance. If it doesn't, take the regular meal. You can choose foods from it and substitute other things from the food supply you are carrying with you. For example, some fresh fruit from home can be substituted for the dessert. Although it is usually recommended that you inject Regular insulin 30 to 60 minutes before eating, in-flight meals are an exception. You should take your insulin only when you see your meal coming down the aisle to avoid unforeseen delays and hypoglycemia.

Be sure to drink plenty of liquids before boarding the flight and drink additional glasses of nonalcoholic liquids each hour you are in the air.

Meal plans and foods. It is important to follow your meal plan even when traveling. An exchange diet lets you substitute many different foods and still adhere to your meal plan. In this country, using exchanges is usually easy. When traveling in foreign countries you may encounter foods that are not familiar to you. Look at ethnic cookbooks before you travel to learn about foods used in the area you will visit. This will help you enjoy meals without difficulty. The usual concern for sanitation is as important for the person with diabetes as for the nondiabetic.

Changes in mealtimes. Carry some food with you. Flights can be delayed and events don't go as scheduled. Depending on your blood glucose level, you need about 10 to 15 grams of carbohydrate, one fruit or one starch/bread, in order to delay your meal by one hour. For meals delayed more than one and a half hours, switch a snack with your meal.

In many foreign countries, it is customary to eat late evening meals. In this case, have your evening snack at the usual evening mealtime and your dinner later. See Chapter 30 for suggestions on how to handle meal and insulin changes.

Another timing problem frequently occurs in Latin countries (Spain, Portugal, and South America). Lunch is often served at 2 p.m. and dinner at 10 p.m. To adjust your meal plan accordingly, begin by having a substantial breakfast. Depending on the amount of exercise and activity planned, you may also need a late morning snack (perhaps your usual afternoon snack) between 11 a.m. and noon. Have lunch at 2 p.m., an early evening snack around 6 p.m. and then dinner at 10 p.m.

With more flexible insulin regimens available today, travel and mealtime changes can be handled in an easier manner. Some insulin regimes or schedules have individuals using a longer acting insulin such as ultra lente and Regular insulin before meals. Another regime calls for NPH and Regular insulin before breakfast, Regular before dinner, and NPH at bedtime. These types of regimes give you more flexibility with your mealtimes when traveling. Ask your doctor or health care team about these possibilities.

Changes in activities. When traveling, you are likely to do a great deal of walking and sightseeing. These activities require changes in your food intake and insulin if they depart from your usual activity patterns.

If you increase your activity level, it is important to include extra snacks or carbohydrate. For moderate exercise, start with an additional fruit or starch/bread exchange. For more strenuous activity of a longer duration you may also need to decrease your insulin dose. See Chapter 33 for suggestions on how to do this. If you have any questions contact your health care team ahead of time.

To add variety, here are some snacks you may find convenient to use while traveling. They can be used when meals are delayed, when driving for extended periods of time, or for increased activity. See Chapter 21 for other ideas.

FOOD	QUANTITY	EXCHANGES
Chips or snack foods	¾ to 1 oz.	1 starch/bread 1–2 fat
Crackers	4 or 5 (1 oz.)	1 starch/bread 0–1 fat
Dried fruit	¼ cup (½ oz.)	1 fruit
Fruit rolls or bars	1 (½ oz.)	1 fruit
Granola bar	1	1 starch/bread 1 fat
Nuts, sunflower seeds	1 oz.	1 med.fat meat 2 fat
Pretzels	¾ oz.	1 starch/bread

Changes in types of food. Visit the library before you travel and check on the cuisine the country has to offer. Or check bookstores for guides to eating out in the country you will be visiting. Food is made of carbohydrates, proteins, and fats wherever you travel! A leafy vegetable, even if grown in Japan instead of in the United States, is still a vegetable exchange. A small to medium fruit is a fruit exchange; starches or grains are starch/bread exchanges; meat, fish, cheese, and eggs are still meat exchanges. And oil is a fat exchange, whether it's sesame or whale oil.

When in doubt about the portion size for a starch/bread or fruit exchange, use ½ cup and you'll be safe. When in doubt about a meat exchange, use 1 ounce for 1 exchange. For a fat exchange, use 1 teaspoon. For mixed dishes, such as casseroles, a one cup portion will be about 2 starch/bread, 2 medium fat meat, and 1 to 2 fat exchanges. A cup of a broth-type soup (noodles, vegetable, rice, and so on) will be one starch/bread exchange and a cup of a cream or bean soup will be one starch/bread and one fat exchange. A bowl of any kind of soup will be 2 starch/breads and 1 to 2 fats.

Translating calories. In some countries you will find "joules" listed on food labels instead of the term calories. Four joules equal one calorie.

Breakfasts are often different. The ever popular continental breakfast usually consists of coffee, rolls, and butter. Breakfasts can be prepared in a hotel room from canned fruit juice or fresh fruit, dry cereal, a bagel, bread, or hard roll, milk, and a beverage. If you plan to prepare your own meals, take along a thermos for milk.

Picnics can be good lunches. For lunch you may enjoy picnicking on food purchased in grocery stores. Try meat and cheese, buns, and fruit. Put them together and you have an inexpensive meal with little or no waste.

Beverages can be a problem in foreign travel. The water often is not safe to drink, and the milk may not be pasteurized. Wine in excess is not a good idea. Sugar-free soft drinks may not be available, and the tea or coffee may be three-fourths cream or milk. You will probably need to use plain coffee or tea, bottled mineral water, wine in moderation, and fruit juice.

Sugar-free soft drinks are becoming more available around the world, but many countries still may not have them available. Many so-called "diabetic" drinks and foods in other countries are sweetened with either fructose or sorbitol. Both these sweeteners have as many calories as sugar. "Un perrier" is a sugarless mineral water with lime flavoring that may be available.

Food and water quality may not be consistent. Precautions with food and water are necessary when traveling outside of the United States to avoid diarrhea and illness. Special care should be taken in South and Central America, Asia, Africa, and Mexico. It is important to know what to do in case of illness.

Know how to treat hypoglycemia. It will be important for you to test your blood glucose when you feel an insulin reaction coming on. Carry a source of glucose so you can treat hypoglycemia (too low a blood glucose level) immediately. Your travel partner should know how to give you glucagon. Glucagon can be used to treat hypoglycemia in a semiconscious or unconscious person, or for persons who refuse or are unable to take food or drink by mouth. Glucagon, like insulin, must be given by injection. Glucagon is now available in a prefilled syringe, but someone with you must know how to give it to you correctly.

Know how to handle illnesses. It is not unusual for individuals to become ill while traveling. Nausea, vomiting, and diarrhea are common problems. If you become ill, it is essential to test your blood glucose a minimum of four times a day (before meals and evening snack) and check urine for ketones. If your blood glucose levels are above 240 mg/dl and urine tests show moderate to large ketones, call a doctor. Besides needing extra Regular insulin, you may have some kind of infection that may need to be treated.

A general guideline for taking extra insulin is to take 10 percent of your total dose as Regular insulin every four to six hours if blood glucose levels are high and ketones are moderate to large. This is in addition to your usual insulin dose. See Chapter 34 for additional information on sick days.

Traveler's diarrhea. A variety of approaches are used in the prevention and treatment of traveler's diarrhea. The most important is the avoidance of food and beverages that are likely to promote the development of diarrhea—milk products such as ice cream and cream sauces; raw or rare meats, poultry, and fish, and soft cheeses; unpeeled fresh fruit; raw vegetables; foods displayed or sold in open markets; poorly refrigerated foods; water and ice cubes. Be sure to seek treatment at the first sign of diarrhea.

And—just a couple more points. Comfortable walking shoes (at least two pairs) should be broken in *before* the trip.

Carry spare prescriptions for prescription drugs and for customs officials an explanatory letter from your physician for insulin syringes. If you are traveling to a non-English-speaking country, carry index cards with emergency phrases in the appropriate language. See some of these at the end of the chapter. If possible, have the name of an English-speaking physician in each city where you will be traveling.

Medical assistance for travelers. If you should need a doctor abroad, the International Association for Medical Assistance to Travelers (IAMAT), a nonprofit organization, has set up centers in 125 countries with English- or French-speaking physicians who are on call 24 hours a day. IAMAT publishes an annual directory of medical centers, along with the names and addresses of associated physicians who have agreed to a set payment schedule for IAMAT cardholders. They also have information on climate, food, and sanitary conditions in countries you may be planning to visit. For more information, write to the IAMAT, 736 Center Street, Lewiston, New York 14092 (716-754-4883); or IAMAT, 188 Nicklin Road, Guelph, Ontario N1H-7L5, Canada.

When traveling abroad, U.S. consuls are available to help you with serious medical, financial, and legal difficulties. Among their many services, U.S. embassies and consulates can:

▲ Help you find medical assistance and inform your family and friends if you are ill or injured.

▲ Assist you in replacing a lost passport or visa.

▲ Arrange to have emergency funds sent by your family, friends, bank, or employer.

▲ Give you information on travel advisories, supply lists of local attorneys, and notarize documents.

Remember, your meal plan travels with you. If you follow your meal plan, anticipate travel situations, and plan carefully, you can have confidence traveling.

Here are some phrases in several foreign languages that may help you when traveling.

▲ German

I am a diabetic.	Ich bin Zuckerkrank. Ich bin Diabetiker (M) Diabetikerin (F).
I am on a special diet.	Ich halte eine Sonderdiät ein.
I need some sugar.	Ich brauche etwas Zucker.
With sugar	Mit Zucker

Without sugar	Ohne Zucker
Sugar added	Zucker hereingestellt
Low calorie	Kalorienarm
No calories	Ohne Kalorien
Low fat	Fettarm
I take daily injections of insulin.	Täglich nehme ich Insulinspritzen.
Please get me a doctor.	Rufen Sie mir bitte einen Arzt.
Sugar or orange juice, please.	Zucker oder Orangensaft, bitte.

▲ Spanish

I am a diabetic.	Yo soy diabético (M) diabética (F).
I am on a special diet.	Estoy a dieta especial.
I need some sugar.	Neccesito azúcar.
Without sugar	Sin azúcar
Sugar added	Con azúcar
Low calorie	Poca calória
No calories	Sin calórias
Low fat	Poca grasa
I take daily injections of insulin.	Tomo inyecciones diarias de insulina.
Please get me a doctor.	Hágame el favor de llamar al médico.
Sugar or a glass of orange juice, please.	Azúcar o un vaso de jugo de naranja, por favor.

▲ French

I am a diabetic.	Je suis diabétique.
I am on a special diet.	Je suis au régime spécial.
I need some sugar.	J'ai besoin de sucre.
Without sugar	Sans sucre
Sugar added	Avec le sucre
I take daily injections of insulin.	Je prends chaque jour une piqûre d'insulin.

Please get me a doctor.	Allez chercher un médecin, s'il vous plâit.
Sugar or orange juice, please.	Sucre ou jus d'orange, s'il vous plâit.

▲ Norwegian

I am a diabetic.	Jeg har sukkersyke.
I am on a special diet.	Jeg har en spesielle diet.
I need some sugar.	Jeg trenger sukker.
With sugar	Med sukker
Without sugar	Utenfor sukker
I take daily injections of insulin.	Jeg tar sproytene daglig.

▲ Italian

I am a diabetic.	Io sono diabetico.
Please get me a doctor.	Per favore chiama un dottore.
Sugar or orange juice, please.	Succhero o succo d'arrangio, per favore.
I take daily injections of insulin.	Predo injectiones de insulin tutti giorni.

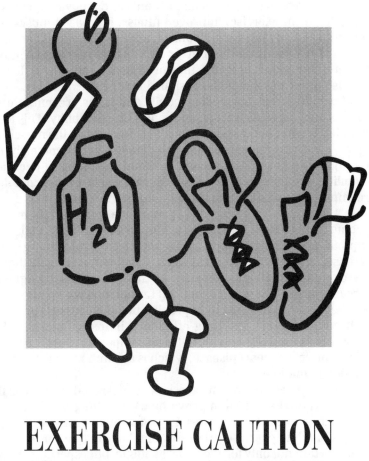

EXERCISE CAUTION
WHEN EXERCISING

Exercise can be beneficial to everyone's health, but it may have some added benefits for you if you have diabetes. Persons with diabetes will experience the same benefits and enjoyment everyone else gains from exercise: improved fitness, increased muscle tone and reduced body fat, weight control, and psychological benefits.

Total fitness includes better flexibility, increased muscle strength and endurance, and improved heart and lung efficiency. Exercise programs should be designed to improve all three.

Flexibility keeps our bodies mobile and helps prevent injury to muscles and joints. As we age, our bodies lose flexibility. This loss of flexibility is what makes people look old. Sometimes the muscle collagen (muscle fibers) in persons with diabetes can become glycosylated (glucose becomes attached to them), resulting in decreased flexibility. Stretching exercises done during warm-up and cool-down are important to help maintain and improve flexibility.

It's no secret that physical appearance improves as muscles become firmer. More importantly, muscle strength and endurance helps us perform our daily tasks with less strain and gives us increased capacity for physical work. It is the muscle cells that use or store carbohydrate. Because of this, exercises designed to increase muscle fibers are beneficial for persons with diabetes and have been shown to assist in improving blood glucose control.

Improved heart and lung efficiency helps us maintain high energy levels for daily activities. It is also important because it helps reduce the risk of heart disease, which is a common long-term complication of diabetes.

Warm-up and cool-down exercises are designed to improve flexibility; aerobic exercises improve heart and lung efficiency; and exercises such as sit-ups, push-ups, and so on are muscle strengthening. Complete exercise programs emphasizing all three aspects are important not only for the general public, but especially for people who have diabetes.

Exercise helps you cope with stress. It builds self-confidence and improves your self-image, especially if you don't think of yourself as athletic yet find you enjoy exercise. You have more energy to do things, are more relaxed, and feel less tense.

Preventing Diabetes!

More importantly, at least three studies monitoring the health of large populations over several years showed that exercise can actually help protect adults predisposed to noninsulin-dependent diabetes from developing it. The major risk factors are a family history of Type II diabetes, obesity, and increasing age.

In a study of 5,990 males over a 14-year period, the risk of developing Type II diabetes fell by six percent for every 500 calorie increase of energy expenditure in leisure time activity in a week. Vigorous activities like running, brisk swimming, cycling, or modern dance were more beneficial than moderate activities like bowling, golf, gardening, or walking.

Another eight-year prospective study of 87,253 women found that women who exercised at least once a week reduced their risk of developing Type II diabetes by about a third. The reduced risk of developing diabetes was true in both obese and normal-weight women and for those who had a family history of diabetes, if they exercised strenuously enough to "work up a sweat" at least once a week.

The same group also reported on 22,271 male physicians studied between 1982 and 1988. In this group regular exercise decreased the incidence of Type II diabetes—the more activity the better. Men who exercised more than five times per week had a 42 percent reduction in risk compared to men who exercised only once a week. But even those who exercised only once a week still had a 23 percent decrease in risk.

The good news is that if you or others in your family are predisposed to develop diabetes, you can do something about it—become involved in a program of regular exercise!

Benefits and Risks of Exercise for Persons Who Have Diabetes

Having diabetes is not a reason to avoid physical activity. On the contrary, diabetes may be another reason to incorporate exercise into your lifestyle. In addition to the benefits listed at the beginning of the chapter, the person with diabetes gains other benefits from exercise.

Regular exercise results in the body cells becoming more sensitive to insulin after exercise, which improves their ability to use and store glucose. Exercise improves risk factors related to heart disease. This includes a lowering of blood cholesterol and triglycerides and an increase in high density cholesterol, the type of cholesterol that protects against heart disease. Exercise also lowers blood pressure.

Exercise combined with a reduction in daily caloric intake will often control noninsulin-dependent or Type II diabetes without the need for other medication. However, physical training, even without weight loss, can help improve the body's ability to use insulin.

Exercise can also pose risks to some persons with diabetes. It is important that you are aware of this and check to see if there are reasons you shouldn't exercise. Before beginning an exercise program, it is important to get your doctor's approval, especially if you are over age 40 or have had diabetes for 10 years or more. Problems such as eye, kidney, or nerve damage may be worsened by inappropriate or strenuous exercise. Nerve damage can blunt or block the body's signals of pain or discomfort from exercise, leading to serious damage before you notice it. Foot problems can develop if proper precautions are not taken.

Exercise also poses some risks to persons with diabetes who take injected insulin or oral hypoglycemic agents (diabetes pills). You need to know how to prevent hypoglycemia (low blood glucose) and to be aware of times when exercise can cause, usually temporarily, hyperglycemia (too high blood glucose).

Getting Started

Before starting any exercise program, be sure your diabetes is under good control. It's important to start slowly and gradually build up endurance.

When you begin an exercise program, the exercise may cause blood glucose levels to change unpredictably. People who exercise regularly usually have fewer blood glucose control problems than those who are just beginning to exercise or who exercise only occasionally.

The key to safe exercise is to monitor your blood glucose before and after exercise. If you are exercising for a long period you should also monitor your blood glucose level during exercise. Discuss your records with your health care team. Together you can develop guidelines for adjusting food intake and insulin.

A good general "rule of thumb" regarding moderate intensity exercise for about one hour concerns blood glucose levels, food intake, and insulin adjustment.

If your blood glucose is less than 100 mg/dl before exercise, eat a pre-exercise snack. See the following chart for snack ideas.

If it is 100 to 150 mg/dl, go ahead and exercise and, if necessary, eat a snack afterwards.

If your blood glucose is greater than 250 mg/dl, check urine for ketones. If ketones are positive, improve blood glucose control by adjusting insulin. Don't exercise until ketones are negative.

▲ PRE- AND POST-EXERCISE SNACKS ▲

FOOD	AMOUNT	CARBO-HYDRATE CONTENT	EXCHANGES
Bagel or English muffin	½	14 gms	1 starch/bread
Graham cracker squares	3	15 gms	1 starch/bread
Snack crackers	4–5	15 gms	1 starch/bread
Muffin	1	17 gms	1 starch/bread, 1 fat
Pretzels	6 3-ring	14 gms	1 starch/bread
Soup (not cream)	1 cup	15 gms	1 starch/bread
Yogurt (plain or sweetened with aspartame)	1 cup	16 gms	1 milk
Apple	1 medium	22 gms	1½ fruit
Banana	1 small	22 gms	1½ fruit
Dried fruit	¼ cup	15 gms	1 fruit
Orange	1 medium	18 gms	1 fruit
Raisins	2 Tbsp	15 gms	1 fruit
Fruit juice	½ cup	15 gms	1 fruit
Gatorade	1 8-oz. cup	12 gms	1 fruit
Exceed: Fluid Replacement and Energy Drink	1 8-oz. cup	17 gms	1 fruit

Before starting any exercise program you need to be aware of the risks of hypoglycemia and hyperglycemia.

Hypoglycemia

Exercise can increase the risk for hypoglycemia, especially if you don't exercise regularly or if you exercise for long periods of time. Hypoglycemia can occur during exercise, usually when you exercise for longer than an hour. Hypoglycemia has been shown to be more common four to 10 hours after exercise than during exercise or even one to two hours after exercise. It can also occur up to 30 hours after vigorous or prolonged exercise or exercise that is done sporadically.

How does this happen? When you begin to exercise, insulin levels drop, but if you take injected insulin your body can't decrease the level of circulating insulin. Just as importantly, exercise causes an increase in "stress hormones"—glucagon, cortisol, growth hormone, adrenaline. As a result of the decrease in insulin and the increase in the stress hormones, the liver releases glucose stored in the liver (glycogen). This keeps blood glucose levels in the normal, or even slightly elevated, range for the first 40 to 60 minutes of exercise, even though exercising muscles may use 20 times more glucose than non-exercising muscles. After about one and a half to two hours of physical activity, in all exercisers, blood glucose levels begin to drop. They may drop somewhat sooner, and can drop dramatically lower in persons who take injected insulin, resulting in hypoglycemia.

After exercise, your blood glucose can continue to drop for two reasons. First, because your body is more sensitive to insulin, it requires less insulin to use or store glucose. Second, your body has to replace the stored carbohydrate (glycogen) used during exercise.

Hypoglycemia can be prevented by increasing food eaten after and/or before exercise or by reducing the dose of insulin acting during the time of activity. See page 314 for general guidelines on how to begin doing this.

Monitor your blood glucose levels at one- or two-hour intervals after—especially strenuous—exercise. It is often more important to eat a small snack after exercising than before. And if you are doing exercise of a long duration, more than one hour, you need to take in some form of carbohydrate during exercise. Incidentally, this is important for all athletes, not just for individuals who have diabetes. Finally, after exercise is completed, don't assume you have exercised safely and disregard making appropriate food or insulin adjustments.

Hyperglycemia

Although low blood glucose levels as a result of exercise are usually the major concern, exercise can at times raise blood glucose levels. One factor that determines the effect exercise has on blood glucose levels is the availability of insulin to muscle cells. With exercise, less insulin is needed, but you do need some insulin. Therefore, if you begin exercising with an insulin deficiency—such as occurs with uncontrolled diabetes—blood glucose levels and ketones can rise.

How does this happen? When blood glucose is high (generally greater than 250 to 300 mg/dl) and urine ketones are moderate to positive, it means not enough insulin is available. You need adequate amounts of insulin available to help the muscle cells use the glucose needed during exercise. Activity is not a replacement for insulin. If blood glucose levels are high, the exercising muscles still need a source of energy and the "stress hormones" cause the liver to release or make more glucose. But because not enough insulin is available, the glucose won't be able to leave the bloodstream to the cells, causing blood glucose to rise during exercise. Meanwhile, the exercising muscles still need a source of energy. Since the extra glucose can't be used, the body responds by releasing fat to be used instead. However, the amount of fat released can be more than the exercising muscles can use, which can lead to an increase in blood and urine ketone levels.

Hyperglycemia is of particular concern when diabetes has been poorly controlled over several days or more. If you start with a blood glucose level greater than 250 or 300 mg/dl, you may find that exercise doesn't decrease it. However, with mild to moderate hyperglycemia (blood glucose levels under 250 to 300 mg/dl), moderate exercise almost always results in a desirable reduction of blood glucose levels.

Exercise of a high intensity can also cause blood glucose levels to be higher after exercise than before. Again, this is probably due to those "stress hormones" causing the liver to release glucose. This can happen even if blood glucose levels are in the normal range before beginning the exercise. High intensity exercise is so strenuous that you become short of breath and have to stop because of exhaustion. Generally, this type of exercise can only be done for short time periods. Examples would be pedaling a bicycle very rapidly, sprinting, climbing stairs quickly, and weight lifting.

Timing of Exercise

The time of day you choose to exercise may also be important. For instance, "morning people" may choose to exercise before breakfast. This is usually a good time to exercise because blood glucose levels tend to be higher during the early morning hours. (However, sometimes the opposite may be true and some people may have lower blood glucose levels before breakfast.) So, if you choose to exercise before breakfast, we suggest you test blood glucose first. If the level is 100 mg/dl or higher, eat or drink 10 to 15 grams of carbohydrate, then exercise. If blood glucose is lower than 100 mg/dl, add another 10 to 15 grams of carbohydrate, wait 10 to 15 minutes, and test again. If it is then above 100 mg/dl, go ahead and exercise. After exercise do another blood glucose test, take your morning insulin, eat breakfast, and enjoy the rest of the day.

Another good time to exercise may be after breakfast (or other meals), since blood glucose levels tend to be the highest during these times. This may be inconvenient because of work or school. But if you can work it out, eat your usual breakfast or meal, exercise, and then have your usual snack. You may find you don't need any extra food.

If you prefer exercising after work or later in the afternoon, do a blood glucose test and follow the recommendations for food adjustment on page 314. Eat the snack before exercising.

If you want to exercise in the evening, take your evening insulin and eat dinner. Wait an hour or so to give your food time to digest, then exercise. (This isn't really necessary, but many persons find they exercise better if they wait awhile after eating.) Test your blood glucose before your evening snack. You may need to add some extra food to that snack, depending on the type and amount of exercise you performed, and the level of your blood glucose. Again, follow the recommendations on page 314. If you exercise later in the afternoon or evening, don't go to bed without a snack. Remember that blood glucose levels continue to drop for hours after exercise.

Guidelines for Safe Exercise

Although studies have not shown that exercise is beneficial in the overall control of blood glucose levels—in fact, blood glucose levels often are harder to control with exercise for persons who take injected insulin—the overall goal is to allow you to begin and/or continue to exercise safely and enjoy the benefits of exercise. For most persons with diabetes, the benefits of exercise far exceed the risks.

You will be your own best teacher when making decisions about blood glucose control during exercise. Blood glucose monitoring is your most effective tool for deciding when and how much to increase food intake or how to reduce insulin dosage appropriately.

Ideally, you would exercise at about the same time each day and at the same level of intensity. For practical reasons, this is rarely possible. You may need to make adjustments, especially in food intake, depending on the time of day you are exercising. Exercise may initially cause blood glucose levels to change unpredictably. Your level of fitness also can affect glucose stability—if you already exercise regularly you will have fewer diabetes control problems than if you are just beginning to exercise or exercise only occasionally.

In general, persons with diabetes tend to overeat before exercise, possibly because of overcautiousness and concern about hypoglycemia, or through a belief that exercise will alleviate the high blood glucose level caused by overeating.

Listed below are general precautions that can help you to exercise safely.

▲ **Be sure you are in good control of your diabetes.** Remember, the effect of exercise will depend on whether enough insulin is available to allow the muscle cells to use glucose for energy.

▲ **Test your blood glucose before and after the exercise session.** If you exercise for a long time, test during the exercise as well. Carefully finding out how exercise affects your blood glucose levels will decrease the risk of hypoglycemia.

▲ **Be aware of the peak times of injected insulin and the excessive lowering of blood glucose levels that exercise may produce at these times.** Regular insulin peaks in three to four hours. NPH or Lente peaks in eight to ten hours. An ideal time to exercise is after a meal, especially after breakfast. If you do exercise when insulin is peaking, be sure to plan for appropriate increases in carbohydrates before or after exercise.

▲ **Continue to monitor blood glucose levels at two hour intervals after strenuous exercise.** Blood glucose can continue to decrease for up to 30 hours after exercise, especially if exercise has been vigorous or prolonged or if exercise is not done regularly.

▲ **Food intake may need to be increased to accommodate activity or exercise.** Regular periods of activity will be planned for in your meal plan. Well-trained persons who regularly exercise usually need less additional food than people who exercise only occasionally. Care should be taken to not eat too much food before exercise.

Extra food eaten before exercise should be in addition to your meal plan. If blood glucose is below 100 mg/dl, eat a snack before exercising. In general, 10 to 15 grams of carbohydrate—one fruit or starch/bread exchange—should be eaten before an hour of moderate exercise, such as tennis, swimming, jogging, cycling, or gardening. For more strenuous activity of a one- to two-hour duration, such as football, hockey, racquetball, basketball, strenuous cycling or swimming, or shoveling heavy snow, 30 to 50 grams of carbohydrate—one-half a meat sandwich with one milk or fruit exchange—may be needed. Mild exercise such as walking a half mile, will probably not require any extra food.

The effect of exercise on blood glucose levels varies greatly. Everyone exercises at different intensities and uses insulin and food differently. The guidelines on page 314, Food Adjustments for Exercise, are only suggestions. They can help you plan food for exercise and make food changes based on your blood glucose level. But, it's still important that you monitor your blood glucose level and adapt these guidelines to your own needs.

Along with food intake, exercisers must remember the need for increased fluid intake. Cool water, sports drinks, or diluted fruit juices are good choices.

▲ **Injection sites are not a major concern, unless the injection is done in a part of your body you will be exercising immediately.** If it's been more than 40 minutes between the injection of Regular insulin and the start of exercise, more than half of the injected insulin will be mobilized from the injection site. Likewise, absorption of intermediate-acting insulin remains unaffected when exercise is begun 1½ hours after an injection. If you exercise immediately after an insulin injection, inject into an area not involved in the exercise, such as the abdomen.

▲ **Be sure to carry identification and a source of readily available carbohydrate with you when you exercise.**

Adjusting Insulin for Extended Exercise

When you exercise strenuously over an extended period, such as all morning, all afternoon, or all day, it may be difficult to avoid low blood glucose by just increasing food intake. In such cases, you can reduce the dose of insulin that will be acting during the time of activity. In effect, the exercise will take the place of the missing insulin and, together with food intake, will keep the blood glucose in the normal range. Use the following guideline to adjust your insulin.

Decrease insulin acting during the exercise time by 10 percent of your total insulin dose. For example:

Insulin dose:	10 Regular	20 NPH before breakfast
	3 Regular	5 NPH before supper
Total:	13 +	25 = 38 units

10 percent of 38 (38 x .10) is 3.8 units, which can be rounded to 4 units. Therefore, you would decrease insulin acting during the time of your activity by 4 units. For instance, Regular insulin acts during the morning hours. For cross-country skiing all morning, you would decrease the morning Regular insulin by 10 percent of the total insulin dose. The morning insulin would then be 6 Regular (10 minus 4) and 20 NPH.

Making Food Adjustments for Exercise: General Guidelines

Type of Exercise and Examples	If Blood Glucose Is:	Increase Food Intake By:	Suggestions of Food to Use
Exercise of short duration and of low to moderate intensity (walking a half mile or leisurely bicycling for less than 30 minutes)	less than 100 mg/dl	10 to 15 gms of carbohydrate per hour	1 fruit or 1 starch/bread exchange
	100 mg/dl or above	not necessary to increase food	
Exercise of moderate intensity (one hour of tennis, swimming, jogging, leisurely bicycling, golfing, etc)	less than 100 mg/dl	25 to 50 gms of carbohydrate before exercise, then 10 to 15 gms per hour of exercise	½ meat sandwich with a milk or fruit exchange
	100 to 180 mg/dl	10 to 15 gms of carbohydrate	1 fruit or 1 starch/bread exchange
	180 to 300 mg/dl	not necessary to increase food	
	300 mg/dl or above	don't begin exercise until blood glucose is under better control	
Strenuous activity or exercise (about one to two hours of football, hockey, racquetball, or basketball; strenuous bicycling or swimming; shoveling heavy snow)	less than 100 mg/dl	50 gms of carbohydrate, monitor blood glucose carefully	1 meat sandwich (2 slices of bread) with a milk and fruit exchange
	100 to 180 mg/dl	25 to 50 gms of carbohydrate, depending on intensity and duration	½ meat sandwich with a milk or fruit exchange
	180 to 300 mg/dl	10 to 15 gms of carbohydrate	1 fruit or 1 starch/bread exchange
	300 mg/dl or above	don't begin exercise until blood glucose is under better control	

Reprinted, with permission, from Diabetes Actively Staying Healthy (DASH): Your Game Plan for Diabetes and Exercise, *by Marion J. Franz, MS, RD and Jane Norstrom, MA. Minneapolis: International Diabetes Center, 1990.*

Intermediate-acting insulin, such as NPH, taken before breakfast acts during the afternoon hours. For canoeing all afternoon, the morning insulin would be 10 Regular and 16 NPH (20 minus 4).

For activity lasting the entire day, such as downhill skiing, the Regular and NPH insulins would each be decreased by 10 percent. This means the morning insulin would be 6 Regular (10 minus 4) and 16 NPH (20 minus 4). On such days you may also need to decrease your insulin at suppertime.

Blood glucose testing before and after physical activity allows you to make adjustments in these general activities. Also make sure that others are aware of your diabetes and know what to do if you need help.

Carbohydrates—The Athlete's Fuel for Exercise

Carbohydrates and fats are the main fuels your body uses for exercise. You don't need to eat fats for fuel, as we all have adequate fat stores—even the very lean athlete. However, we do need to eat carbohydrates, because our body has only a limited capacity to store carbohydrate as glycogen in muscles and the liver. Glycogen from muscles and liver releases glucose, a fuel used for exercise.

Eating a diet that contains adequate amounts of carbohydrates on a regular basis promotes glycogen storage. But there are times before, during, and after exercise when extra carbohydrates are needed for all athletes, especially athletes who have diabetes.

Before. Although eating carbohydrates on a regular basis is beneficial to exercise performance, eating carbohydrates immediately before exercising hasn't been shown to have much effect on how well you exercise. During the first 40 or so minutes of exercise our bodies use glucose from the carbohydrates stored as glycogen in the muscle and liver.

But if you have diabetes, it is a good idea to eat a small amount of carbohydrate before you exercise, especially if you are exercising at peak times of insulin action. A simple pre-exercise snack of 10 to 15 grams of carbohydrate won't elevate blood glucose levels very much, but might prevent hypoglycemia, especially if your blood glucose levels were in the process of dropping before you started to exercise. Take care not to overeat and follow the suggestions given earlier in the chapter.

During exercise. Studies have shown that all athletes are able to exercise longer if they eat some form of carbohydrate during exercise, especially when exercising for longer than an hour at a time. Whenever anyone does moderately intense exercise for more than one-and-a-half hours, blood glucose levels begin to drop. If you have diabetes, your blood glucose levels may begin to drop sooner and continue to drop too low if you don't take in some form of carbohydrate. Ingesting 10 to 15 grams of carbohydrate every hour during a long event can be very important. For very intense or competitive activities, such as marathons, you may need 10 to 15 grams of carbohydrate every 30 minutes. At this point in your training program, you have probably made significant reductions in your dose of insulin as well.

For up to 40 minutes of exercise, plain water is the best beverage for all athletes. After that, carbohydrates are needed to delay the onset of fatigue. If the carbohydrate is too concentrated, the body cannot absorb it rapidly. Concentrated carbohydrates can also lead to stomach cramping or discomfort, nausea, bloating, and/or diarrhea. Sports drinks or Gatorade have been shown to be beneficial during exercise because they are diluted carbohydrates (less than 10 percent sugar) and therefore are emptied from the stomach and absorbed from the intestine as rapidly as water. They provide fuel, help control body temperature, and can help keep blood glucose levels in an appropriate range. Fruit juices and regular soft drinks are about 12 percent or more carbohydrate, so they need to be diluted with an equal amount of water (½ cup juice, ½ cup water) in order to be absorbed more quickly.

After exercise. For all athletes, eating carbohydrates within two hours and preferably within 20 minutes after exercise is important. Glycogen used during exercise must be replaced; at this time the body is more sensitive to insulin and more carbohydrate will be stored as glycogen. Eat at least 0.7 grams of carbohydrate per pound of body weight shortly after exercise and again in 60 minutes. This would be about 75 grams of carbohydrate.

If you have diabetes, you must replace carbohydrate after exercise to prevent delayed hypoglycemia, which may occur several hours, and even 24 to 30 hours, after you exercise.

Fluids. Dehydration (lack of fluids) can contribute to fatigue, heat cramps, heat exhaustion, and even heat stroke. Proper hydration is essential if you are to perform to the best of your ability. Loss of body fluids in sweat makes it harder to regulate your body temperature. Losing as little as two percent of your body weight through sweat impairs your ability to exercise. For a 150-pound person, this would only be a loss of 3 pounds. Marathon runners might lose 6 to 8 percent of their body weight, while more moderate activity can lead to losses of 2 to 4 percent. Dehydration is a major limiting factor to how well and how long you are able to exercise.

It is important that you replace fluid losses. Don't wait until you feel thirsty—by then, you are already dehydrated. For every pound of weight lost during exercise, you need to drink two cups of water. Athletes with diabetes often become so preoccupied with eating carbohydrates they forget that the first nutrient needed by all exercisers is water.

You also need to be sure to drink plenty of fluids before exercise. Two hours before an event, drink 2 to 3 cups of cold water; 10 to 15 minutes before, drink 1 to 2 cups more. Drink small amounts, ½ to 1 cup, at 15- to 20-minute intervals during exercise, especially during warm weather.

Meals on days of athletic events. On the day of competition, a breakfast of toast, juice or fruit, and cereal with skim milk is a good choice. A turkey or other lean meat sandwich, broth-type soup, skim milk, and fruit make up a good lunch.

A pregame meal should be eaten one to three hours before the event. The meal should contain mainly carbohydrate, some protein, but little fat. Lean meat (fish or poultry), potatoes or other starch without butter or gravy, vegetables, bread or rolls with no butter, salad without dressing, fruit, and skim milk can be on the menu. Three to 4 cups of fluid should be included with the meal. Continue to drink fluids up to the time of competition. Additional carbohydrates, such as fruit or fruit juice, should be eaten 20 minutes before the event.

These nutrition guidelines can help you get started, but each individual athlete varies in his or her response to training and physical activity. Be responsive to the signals your body provides and become an expert in interpreting these signals.

Exercise and Noninsulin-Dependent Diabetes

Routine exercise helps in the management of Type II diabetes because working muscles use and store glucose more effectively. Research has shown that a combination of physical training and meal planning produces a greater increase in insulin sensitivity than meal planning alone. Even a single bout of exercise has been shown to improve blood glucose levels for up to 12 to 16 hours later.

However, the benefits of exercise on blood glucose levels are short-lived. Exercise must be done regularly for it to improve blood glucose control. For sustained improvement of blood glucose control, exercise must be performed three or more times a week. The more you exercise, the more improvement you will see in your diabetes control. Studies show that frequently repeated activity is more important than high-intensity (exercise done to the point of exhaustion) activity.

Exercise can also be a way to burn excess calories and help with weight loss. About 3,500 calories are stored in one pound of fat. Therefore, to lose one pound of fat, you must (1) reduce your calorie intake by 3,500 calories, (2) increase your activity level by 3,500 calories, or (3) do a combination of both. Decreasing your calorie intake by 500 calories a day and adding 250 calories of activity gives you a deficit of 5,250 calories in one week, or a loss of 1½ pounds of fat.

The chart, Using 250 Calories, will give you some idea of how much exercise is needed to burn 250 calories. These calorie estimates are general averages; how many calories you actually burn depends on how hard and how skillfully you perform the activity. As you can see, it takes a significant amount of exercise to lose weight by exercise alone, so you also have to watch what you eat!

USING 250 CALORIES
▲ THROUGH EXERCISE ▲

	MINUTES NEEDED TO BURN 250 CALORIES		
	129 lbs (54.5 kg)	150 lbs (68 kg)	220 lbs (90 kg)
Activity			
Aerobic dancing (doesn't include warm-up and cool-down)	27	22	16
Bicycling (6 mph)	71	57	43
(12 mph)	27	22	16
Bowling	100	83	71
Calisthenics	69	56	42
Dancing (slow)	89	71	54
(fast)	27	22	16
Golf (walking with bag)	54	43	32
Running or jogging			
(5 mph)	34	27	20
(7.5 mph)	24	19	14
(10 mph)	18	15	11
Skiing (cross-country)	38	31	23
Racquetball	42	34	25
Swimming			
(fast, freestyle)	36	29	22
Tennis (singles)	42	34	25
(doubles)	71	57	43
Walking (3 mph)	74	58	44
(4 mph)	49	39	29
(up stairs)	32	26	19

Guidelines for Exercising Safely

If you take insulin or diabetes pills to help control blood glucose levels, be aware of the precautions discussed earlier in the chapter. However, since your body is still producing insulin, your blood glucose levels will not be as unstable with exercise as those in persons whose pancreas is no longer producing any insulin. You will not generally need to eat extra food before or after exercise.

▲ **It's very important to start slowly and gradually increase the amount of time you exercise each day until you reach your desired time goal.** The most efficient way to burn fat is to exercise continuously for at least 20 to 30 minutes (long duration) at a perceived exertion level of "somewhat strong" (see chart below), which results in no shortness of breath (low intensity). This type of exercise uses stored fat as the major energy source. Exercise under two to three minutes (short duration) that causes shortness of breath (high intensity) uses stored carbohydrate as the major energy source and is not as helpful for weight control.

▲

Perceived Exertion Scale

Rating	Description
0	Nothing at all
0.5	Very, very weak
1.0	Very weak
2	Weak
3	Moderate
4	Somewhat strong
5	Strong
6	
7	Very strong
8	
9	
10	Very, very strong
	Maximal

Reprinted, with permission, from Guidelines for Exercise Testing and Prescription, *Figure 2–3, by American College of Sports Medicine. Philadelphia: Lea & Febiger, 1986:23.*

▲ **Put your emphasis on aerobic exercise (exercise that is lower in intensity and longer in time).** This type of exercise burns calories more effectively.

▲ **For weight control, do aerobic exercise for at least 25 to 30 minutes, five to six days a week.** Begin gradually, with five- to 10-minute exercise sessions. The goal is to burn 250 to 300 calories per session.

▲ **Exercise should be low-impact to prevent injury to bones and joints.** Low-impact exercises are done with at least one foot touching the floor at all times. There is no jumping or jarring to put stress on the joints. Exercise recommended for weight loss includes brisk walking, swimming, bicycling, and low-impact aerobic dance.

▲ **Muscle strengthening exercises can also be helpful for improving blood glucose levels.** This increases muscle mass and muscles use more glucose than fat does. However, avoid strenuous weight lifting and isometric exercises. They increase blood pressure and cause or aggravate kidney and eye problems.

▲ **Support from family or friends is important.** It's easy to get discouraged when improvement comes much slower than you would like. That's why a group exercise class can be especially helpful.

▲ **Choose activities you enjoy.** Vary your activities.

▲ **Exercise at a time of day that is best for you.** You will be more likely to stick with it.

The Bottom Line—

Exercise should be fun. Regular exercisers stick with it because they enjoy it. It may take time to develop this attitude toward exercising, but eventually the rewards will present themselves—"the sound of cheering from within"—and *not* exercising will become unthinkable.

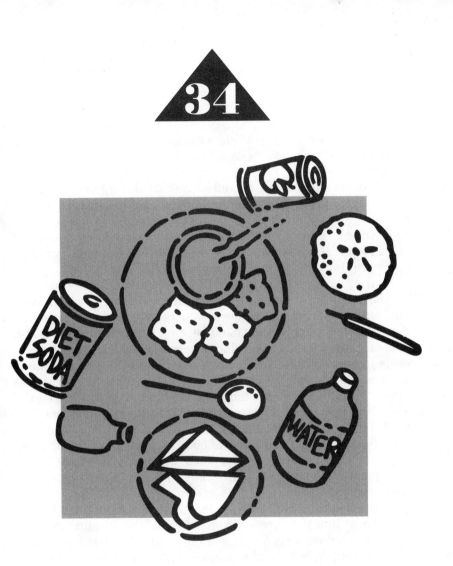

MEAL PLANNING
DURING A BRIEF
ILLNESS

Colds, fever, flu, nausea, vomiting, diarrhea—these are all common illnesses that may cause special problems for people with diabetes.

Diabetes can get out of control quickly during illness. Fever, dehydration (loss of body fluid), infection, and the stress of illness can all trigger the release of "stress" hormones (glucagon, epinephrine and norepinephrine, cortisol, and growth hormone) that raise blood glucose levels. As a result of this, the body requires more insulin.

During stress, such as illness, these "stress" hormones normally provide the brain and muscles with sources of energy by increasing the levels of glucose and ketones. In persons who do not have diabetes this does not get out of hand because additional insulin is also released, which keeps blood glucose levels normal. Insulin also prevents the uncontrolled breakdown of fat and excessive buildup of ketones in the blood. For individuals who have diabetes, the actions of the "stress hormones" tend to be unchecked or poorly checked because of the lack of effective insulin. When the body does not have the help of sufficient insulin, the ketones build up in the blood and then "spill" into the urine so the body can get rid of them. When present in large amounts in the blood, ketones (which are types of acids) cause ketoacidosis. Ketoacidosis, if untreated, can lead to coma and even death.

Persons with insulin-dependent diabetes must have insulin throughout illness to prevent ketoacidosis. This insulin is needed even if the individual is eating less than usual as a result of nausea and vomiting. In fact, insulin requirements usually increase during illness, because "stress hormones" raise blood glucose levels more than eating does.

People with Type II diabetes who take insulin or diabetes pills (oral hypoglycemic agents) to help control blood glucose also must continue taking their medication. Even people with Type II diabetes who are not taking insulin or diabetes pills may temporarily need insulin to control blood glucose during times of illness.

During a brief illness you can manage your food and insulin balance by following the guidelines listed below. These guidelines apply to mild, one-day illnesses. If you are ill for longer than one day, call your health care team for additional advice.

Guidelines

▲ **When you are ill, it is very important to take your usual dose of insulin.** Your need for insulin continues or increases during illness. Never omit your insulin. If in doubt, begin by taking your usual amount of insulin. If you normally don't use Regular insulin, have a vial of Regular insulin on reserve to use during illness as directed.

▲ **If you take diabetes pills, take your usual dose, unless you are vomiting.** Once you are able to keep fluids down and can eat food again, take your pill.

▲ **Monitor your blood glucose and test urine for ketones at least four times a day—before each meal and at bedtime.** This may need to be done more often when you are ill. Even with blood glucose monitoring, you still need to test urine for ketones. If your blood glucose reading is higher than 240 mg/dl, it is especially important to test a urine sample for ketones. The combination of a high blood glucose level and moderate to large ketones in the urine is a danger signal. Call your health care team if this happens.

▲ **If you can't eat your regular foods, replace them with carbohydrates in the form of liquids or soft foods.** See examples listed on the chart Foods to Replace Meals During Brief Illness. Eat at least 50 grams of carbohydrates every three to four hours, especially if your blood glucose level is 240 mg/dl or less. This will provide some readily available sugar so your body won't have to burn fat for energy, which produces ketones. It will also prevent blood glucose levels from dropping too rapidly. It's important to eat these foods in small, frequent feedings. The sick day menu shown will give you an idea of when and what to eat.

▲

Sick Day Menu

	Food	Carbohydrate Content
8:00 A.M.	1 slice toast	15 gm
Spread throughout morning	12 oz sugar-containing soft drink	30 gm
Noon	1 cup soup	15 gm
	6 saltine crackers	15 gm
Spread throughout afternoon	12 oz sugar-containing soft drink	30 gm
6:00 P.M.	½ cup Jello	20 gm
Spread throughout evening	12 oz sugar-containing soft drink	30 gm
		155 gms

If your blood glucose levels are higher than 240 mg/dl, don't be too concerned if you are unable to eat the entire 50 grams of carbohydrate. However, be sure to continue to drink liquids, especially those that don't contain calories, such as water, broth, diet soft drinks, and tea.

▲ **Drink a large glass of calorie-free liquid every hour.** During illness body fluids and minerals are lost rapidly and must be replaced to prevent dehydration. This is especially true if you have fever, diarrhea, or vomiting. If you feel nauseated or are vomiting, take small sips of liquid—one or two tablespoons every 15 to 30 minutes—and call your health care team.

"Drink fluids and take aspirin"—the usual advice during illness—is also helpful for adults with diabetes. The aspirin reduces fever and controls secretion of the stress-produced hormones. Children should use a pain reliever such as Tylenol.

▲ **Call your health care team if:**
- You can't keep any liquids or carbohydrates down for more than eight hours.
- You are vomiting or have diarrhea.
- You are spilling ketones in your urine.
- You begin to breathe rapidly, become drowsy, or lose unconsciousness.

▲ **When illness subsides, return to your regular meal plan and usual insulin schedule.** When you are well again and you need help with continued insulin adjustments, call or visit your health care team.

The foods listed in the following table contain carbohydrates and are often easily tolerated by most people during a brief illness. Choose foods or beverages that you feel you can tolerate when ill. Remember, you want to take in about 50 grams of carbohydrate every three to four hours or for each missed meal. This should be done in small, frequent feedings.

FOODS TO REPLACE MEALS
▲ DURING BRIEF ILLNESS ▲

The following foods are often tolerated by people during periods of illness. To replace 10 or 15 grams of carbohydrate, use any of the following foods in the amount indicated.

Foods Containing 10 Grams Carbohydrate	Quantity
Carbonated beverages containing sugar (ginger ale, cola)*	½ cup (4 oz)
Popsicle	½ twin bar
Corn syrup or honey	2 tsp
Granulated sugar	2½ tsp (5 small cubes)
Sweetened gelatin (Jello®)	¼ cup
Coke syrup	1 tbsp (½ oz)

Foods Containing 15 Grams Carbohydrate	Quantity
Orange juice, grapefruit juice	½ cup
Grape juice, apple juice	⅓ cup
Ice cream	½ cup
Cooked cereal	½ cup
Sherbet	¼ cup
Jello	⅓ cup
Broth-based soups, reconstituted with water	1 cup
Cream soups	1 cup
Carbonated beverages containing sugar (ginger ale, cola)*	¾ cup (6 oz)
Milkshake	¼ cup
Milk	1½ cups (10 oz)
Eggnog, commercial	½ cup
Tapioca pudding	⅓ cup
Custard	½ cup
Yogurt, plain	1 cup
Toast	1 slice
Saltine crackers	6

*Soft drinks opened and left at room temperature for a few minutes to allow for "decarbonation" will usually be better tolerated.

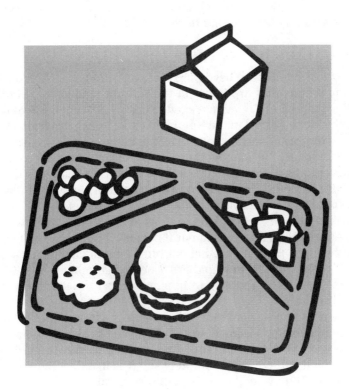

SCHOOL LUNCH— EXCHANGE THOSE MENUS

School bells signal the start of a new school year. An area of concern for students with diabetes is the lunch program. Should they carry a bag lunch or eat the school lunch?

School Lunch Programs

Today most schools are becoming more nutrition conscious and are offering menus that are lower in fat, sodium, and sugar. Students who have diabetes are encouraged to eat school lunches whenever possible. Meals served in the National School Lunch Program (NSLP) are an example of portion control and introduce students to a wider variety of foods. Putting together an appropriate meal from cafeteria line options is good practice in food decision making for the student with diabetes. There are, however, several considerations that must be kept in mind by the student who has diabetes.

It is important to check the menus ahead of time to determine if the entire menu may be used or if part of it should be replaced by foods brought from home. School lunch menus are usually published weekly in local newspapers. Encourage schools to post last-minute changes in the school lunchroom, so the student can be alerted to them.

The occasional appearance of sweet desserts in the school lunch can be a problem. A cookie or a plain piece of cake, without icing, can be used as a starch/bread exchange. However, fresh fruit or fruit canned without the addition of sugar is usually recommended for dessert. It may need to be brought from home.

Ninety percent of the schools in the United States participate in the National School Lunch Program, which is operated by the Food and Nutrition Service of the U.S. Department of Agriculture. Meal patterns required by NSLP regulations are designed to provide students with about one-third of the daily nutrients they need. A school lunch must consist of five different food items from four food component groups:

   2 oz. serving of meat or meat alternative (cheese, soy, peanut butter, vegetable protein products).

   2 or more servings of vegetables or fruits or both.

   1 serving of whole grain or enriched bread or alternative (noodles, pasta, rice, tortillas); 8 servings per week.

1 serving of ½ pint of low-fat milk (½, 1, 1½, or 2 percent fat) or whole milk. Schools must offer both to students.

The required minimum amounts of each item served vary according to the age or grade group. Since younger children are not always able to eat the amount specified, regulations permit serving lesser amounts. For teenagers, regulations call for the serving of larger amounts of selected foods. Senior high students can choose at least three of the five food items served. This is called Offer Versus Serve. Additionally, junior high, middle, and elementary schools may also choose to participate in this program. This allows these students to also choose three or four of the five menu items. However, although not required to do so, some cafeteria personnel will make substitutions, such as fresh fruit in place of a sweet dessert, if they are aware that a student has diabetes.

To incorporate school lunch, the following meal plan for students with diabetes usually works well:

2–4 starch/bread exchanges	1 fruit exchange
2 meat exchanges	1 milk exchange
1–2 vegetable exchanges	2–3 fat exchanges

The meal plan will vary with the age of the student. For the younger child (kindergarten through second grade) usually 2 starch/bread exchanges, 1–2 meat and a smaller number of fat exchanges will be sufficient. Older students (particularly high school boys) will require additional starch/bread and perhaps meat, milk, and fat exchanges, since these are usually available for seconds. Weight-watching teens may need fewer exchanges, especially fat exchanges. If the food service at school is aware of the food exchanges in the student's meal plan, they are usually able to serve portions that will fulfill the student's need.

In planning school lunches remember that *when* lunch is eaten can be as crucial as *what* is eaten. Secondly, lunch should be eaten at approximately the same time every day—sometime between 11:30 a.m. and 1:00 p.m. is usually best. If the school lunch is served earlier, the student may need two afternoon snacks—perhaps at around 2:00 or 2:30 and again around 4:00. If lunchtime is after 1:00 p.m. a mid-morning snack is necessary.

SAMPLE MENUS

▲ School Lunches ▲

The following are some examples of menus, menus with substitutions and inappropriate school lunch menus.

Food	Exchanges
Pizza	2 starch/bread
	2 meat
	1–2 fat
Hard roll/butter	1 starch/bread
	1 fat
Tossed salad	1 vegetable
Dressing	1–2 fat
Fresh fruit	1 fruit
Low-fat milk	1 milk

Total: 3 starch/bread, 2 meat, 1 vegetable, 1 fruit, 1 milk, 3–4 fat exchanges

Food	Exchanges
Barbecue beef on bun	1½ starch/bread
	2 meat
Tater tots	1½ starch/bread
	1–2 fat
Carrots	1 vegetable
Cookie	1 starch/bread
	1 fat
Low-fat milk	1 milk

Total: 4 starch/bread, 2 meat, 1 vegetable, 1 milk, 2–3 fat exchanges

Need: 1 fruit exchange (or substitute 1 starch/bread for the fruit exchange)

Food	Exchanges
Tacos	2 starch/bread
	2 meat
Lettuce/tomato	1 vegetable
Mexicali corn	1 starch/bread
Fruit cup	1 fruit
Low-fat milk	1 milk

Total: 3 starch/bread, 2 meat, 1 vegetable,
1 fruit, 1 milk exchange

Menu with Modification

Food	Exchanges
Beef ravioli	2 starch/bread
	2 meat
Garlic bread	1 starch/bread
	1–2 fat
Green beans	1 vegetable
Brownie	(substitute fresh fruit)
Low-fat milk	1 milk

Total: 3 starch/bread, 2 meat, 1 vegetable,
1 milk, 2–3 fat exchanges

Need: 1 fruit exchange for substitution

Inappropriate Menu

Food	Problem
Fried chicken	high-fat preparation
Home fries	high fat
Corn on cob/butter	OK
Peaches in heavy syrup	sugared fruit
2% chocolate milk	sugared milk

School Breakfast Programs

Some schools also participate in the School Breakfast Program (SBP). If they do, a complete school breakfast now consists of:

1 serving of ½ pint milk.

1 serving of fruit or vegetable or both, or fruit or vegetable juice.

2 servings of bread or a bread alternative (bread, biscuits, rolls, muffins, cornbread, or cereal) or meat or a meat alternative (1 oz. meat, poultry, fish or cheese; ½ egg; 2 Tbsp. peanut butter) or one serving from each group.

Schools also have the Offer Versus Serve option for school breakfasts. Students must then be offered all four required food items and are permitted to refuse one food item from any component they do not plan to eat.

Snacks

Snacks are very important for the student with diabetes. Food is divided into a series of meals and snacks to match the time actions of insulins. Morning snacks are usually light and may consist of a fruit or starch/bread exchange and/or one-half pint of milk. Some students may have a small snack in the middle of the afternoon school session followed by a snack after arriving home. Snacks may need to be larger on days when the student has a physical education class or active recess period. Depending on the time of gym or recess snacks may be eaten before or after the activities.

Snacks may consist of fresh fruit, dried fruit, crackers, milk, a half or whole sandwich or some form of convenience food. Students should be allowed to eat as inconspicuously and with as little fuss as possible. See Chapter 21 for other snack ideas.

Students with diabetes are encouraged to participate in school sports programs. This will require eating a substantial snack before practice and games. They may also need additional carbohydrates during practice or during games.

School Parties

School parties frequently pose a problem for students with diabetes because of the amount of sweets served. However, some of these foods may be used as part of a meal plan. The following are examples of party foods that may be counted as one starch/bread exchange plus one to two fat exchanges.

▲

Food	Quantity
Cookie, 3" diameter	1
Cookie, 1¾" diameter	2
Plain cake	1 piece, 2" square
Cupcake, without frosting	1
Angel food cake	1 small piece
Frozen yogurt	1/3 cup
Ice cream	1/2 cup
Ice milk	1/2 cup

Sugar free soft drinks or Kool-Aid sweetened with artificial sweeteners may be used as a free food. Dietetic hard candies can be used in limited quantities.

Other dietetic food products, such as the chocolate candies, cakes, ice cream or cookies, are not recommended. They are usually higher in calories than the foods they are replacing.

Students and parents are encouraged to educate teachers and other school personnel about diabetes. The more knowledgeable school personnel are, the more cooperative and helpful they can be.

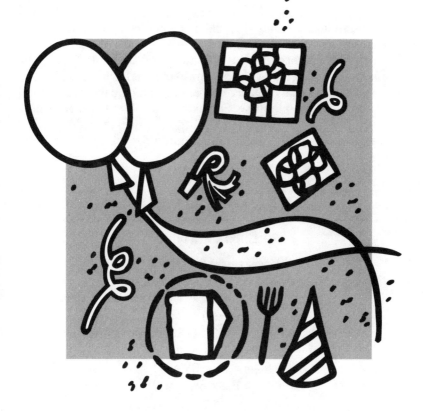

CHILDREN'S PARTIES

Birthday and other parties are a time of added excitement and exercise for young children. The child with diabetes may need additional food because of the increased activity. The person giving the party should know that the child has diabetes and should be told how to recognize a reaction and what to do in case of one.

Serving food before the activities and games is helpful. Then the extra food or special foods can be compensated for by exercise.

For a birthday party you can use an angel food cake frosted with a low-calorie whipped topping. Sprinkle with colored sugarless beverage base (such as unsweetened Kool-Aid powder) and add candles!

Here is a workable and popular menu for a child's birthday party.

SAMPLE MENU

▲ Child's Party ▲

Hamburgers in Small Buns
(Meat and Starch/Bread Exchanges)
Carrot Sticks, Celery Sticks and Dill Pickles
(Free)
Unsweetened Fruit in Artificially Sweetened Gelatin
(Fruit Exchange)
Angel Food Cake
(Starch/Bread Exchange)
Ice Cream, Ice Milk or Frozen Yogurt
(Starch/Bread and Fat Exchanges)

Other party menu ideas include:

▲ **Pizza Spinners:** Begin with one 7½ ounce can refrigerator biscuits. On a baking sheet, flatten out each biscuit with fingers until doubled in size. Spread 2 teaspoons pizza sauce on each biscuit. Sprinkle with 1 tablespoon ham and 1 tablespoon shredded part-skim mozzarella cheese. Bake at 400° for 8 to

10 minutes. Each spinner equals 1 starch/bread and ½ medium-fat meat exchange.

▲ **Chocolate Arrows:** Melt 1 teaspoon margarine and 1 tablespoon mini-semisweet chocolate chips together in a small pan over low heat, stirring constantly. Remove from heat when melted. Dunk ends of 32 pretzel sticks in chocolate. Put on rack to cool. Eight arrows equal ½ starch/bread and 1 fat exchange.

▲ **Frozen Juice Cubes:** Freeze fruit juice in an ice cube tray. Crush cubes in blender or food processor for fruit slush or snow cones. Four cubes equal 1 fruit exchange.

▲ **Frozen Bananas:** Peel and cut the banana in half crosswise. Slide popsicle stick into cut end of banana half, roll in wheat germ, stand in jar, place in freezer. One equals 1 fruit exchange.

▲ **Banana Chips:** Slice 4 small bananas and dip into lemon juice. Place on oiled sheet in a single layer. Bake at 175° for 2 to 3 hours, until golden. Store in an airtight container. One fourth of the recipe equals 1½ fruit exchange.

▲ **Pink Perfect Popcorn:** Keep 6 cups of popped popcorn warm in oven. In small saucepan over low heat, melt 1½ tablespoons margarine. Cool slightly. Quickly stir in 1 teaspoon sugar-free strawberry flavored gelatin and immediately pour over popcorn, tossing to coat all pieces. Once cup equals 1 starch/bread and 1 fat exchange.

▲ **Purple Ice:** Combine ¾ cup grape juice, ½ cup vanilla ice milk, and ¾ cup plain nonfat yogurt in blender. Blend until smooth. Pour over ice into 2 glasses. One cup (½ recipe) equals 1 fruit and 1 milk or 1 starch/bread exchange and 1 fruit.

▲ **Sugar-Free Popsicles:** Combine one package of sugar-free gelatin, one package of Kool-Aid, one tablespoon artificial sweetener, two cups of boiling water, and two cups of cold water. Freeze in ice cube trays with sticks. Calories are negligible; free exchange.

For more ideas for party snacks see *Joy of Snacks* by Nancy Cooper.

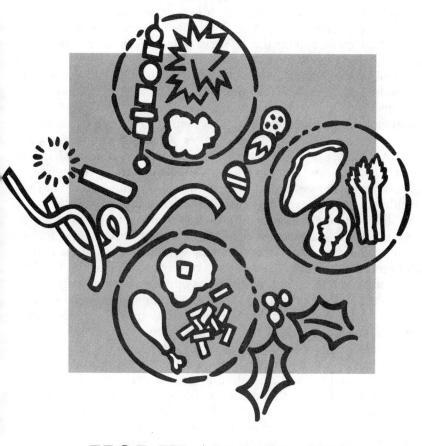

HOLIDAY MENUS

Sociable persons are often hosts or guests, and diabetes should not curb sociability. If a party is given at home by the person with diabetes, there should be few problems since he or she can control the menu and the time of serving, but information about holiday and party foods can also help.

For persons taking insulin, timing of meals on holidays can be a problem. For example, if the family chooses to have the holiday meal at 2 or 3 p.m. and you are scheduled to eat at 12 noon and 6 p.m., what can you do to enjoy the holiday festivities with your family or friends? Begin by having the exchanges of your afternoon snack at 12 noon. Then, at 2 or 3 p.m. have the exchanges of your lunch meal plan. Chances are that you will probably use part of your dinner meal plan exchanges at that time as well. Do save a portion of the evening meal plan exchanges to eat at the routine supper hour.

Making these changes will probably throw your blood glucose tests off for that day because you may be testing closer to mealtimes than you normally do. But by knowing what has affected the blood glucose tests, you don't need to make any changes in the insulin program. Keep in mind that dividing your meal plan into different size meals and snacks won't get you into trouble as long as the total carbohydrate and calorie intake for the day (preferably for each four- to six-hour period) remains the same. For persons taking insulin, delaying meals will cause problems! One of the factors that determines how much insulin is needed in a day is the total number of calories eaten, and this should remain constant. Above all, remember that these changes should be reserved for very special occasions!

The same principle applies to days when you need to have your larger meal at noon instead of in the evening. For that day exchange your noon and evening meal plans.

Meal planning by the individual with diabetes depends on a certain amount of self-control as well as adequate information. With this combination, you can enjoy a normal social life and even "have a ball!"

These menu suggestions may help your holiday planning. Recipes for the starred items are found in Chapter 38. The number of exchanges you count in your meal plan will depend upon the amount you decide to eat.

SAMPLE MENU

▲ Thanksgiving ▲

Spicy Tomato Cocktail*
(Free)

Roast Turkey	**Dressing**
(Meat Exchange)	(Starch/Bread and Fat Exchanges)
Gravy	**Mashed Potatoes**
(Fat Exchange)	(Starch/Bread Exchange)

Cauliflower Supreme*
(Vegetable, Fruit, and Fat Exchanges)

Cranberry-Celery Salad*
(Free)

Rolls	**Margarine**
(Starch/Bread Exchange)	(Fat Exchange)

Low-Cal Pumpkin Pie* with Low-Calorie Whipped Topping
(Starch/Bread and Fat Exchanges)

Coffee	**Milk**
(Free)	(Milk Exchange)

SAMPLE MENU

▲ Christmas ▲

Sparkling Sugar-Free Punch*
(Free)

Fresh Vegetable Slices
(Free)
with

Cottage Cheese Dip
(Cottage cheese pureed in blender with
onions, parsley, and seasonings)
(Meat Exchange)

Roast Beef Au Jus
(Meat Exchange)

Browned Potatoes   **Green Beans Oregano***
(Starch/Bread and Fat Exchanges)   (Vegetable Exchange)

Garden Green Salad with Low-Calorie Dressing
(Free)

Rolls   **Margarine**
(Starch/Bread Exchange)   (Fat Exchange)

Flaming Cherries Jubilee*
(Fruit, Starch/Bread, and Fat Exchanges)

Coffee   **Milk**
(Free)   (Milk Exchange)

SAMPLE MENU

▲ Easter ▲

Baked Ham
(Baste with sugar-free ginger ale)
(Meat Exchange)

Potato Soufflé*   **Fresh Asparagus Spears**
(Starch/Bread and Fat Exchanges)   (Vegetable Exchange)

Carrot Orange Toss*
(Fruit and Vegetable Exchanges)

Rolls   **Margarine**
(Starch/Bread Exchange)   (Fat Exchange)

Strawberry Trifle*
(Fruit and Starch/Bread Exchanges)

Coffee   **Milk**
(Free)   (Milk Exchange)

SAMPLE MENU

▲ Fourth of July ▲

Backyard Barbecue

Chicken on the Grill   **Potato Salad**
(Meat Exchange)   (Starch/Bread and Fat Exchanges)

Grilled Vegetable Kabobs
(Cherry Tomatoes, Zucchini, Mushroom, Small Onion)

Relishes
(Vegetable Exchanges)

Rolls   **Margarine**
(Starch/Bread Exchange)   (Fat Exchange)

Marshmallow Crispies*
(Fruit Exchange)
OR

Angel Macaroons*
(Starch/Bread and Fat Exchanges)

Watermelon
(Fruit Exchange)

Low-Calorie Lemonade   **Sugar-Free Soda Pop**
(Free)   (Free)

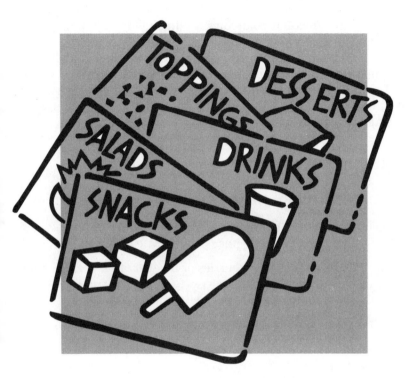

SELECTED RECIPES

This guide for using the exchange system for meal planning was not designed as a recipe book, but a sampling of especially helpful recipes is included.

Recipe modification guidelines are included in Chapter 23 and will help you modify your favorite recipes. These guidelines help to reduce fat, sugar, and calories. Chapter 28 contains guidelines to help you convert your favorite recipes into exchanges.

These first recipes can be used as delicious toppings on pancakes or French toast. Add a dab of plain, low-fat yogurt and you have an attractive serving.

▲

Strawberry and Blueberry Topping

2 cups fresh or frozen (without sugar) strawberries or blueberries
2 tsp. undiluted frozen apple juice concentrate (thawed)

Combine ½ cup of sliced strawberries or blueberries and 2 tsp. apple juice concentrate in a blender; process to a smooth sauce. Pour over remaining sliced strawberries or blueberries.

Yield:	4 servings	Serving size: ¾ cup
Per serving of strawberries:		
Calories:		56
Carbohydrate:		14 gms
Sodium:		1 mg
Exchanges:		1 fruit
Per serving of blueberries:		
Calories:		64
Carbohydrate:		16 gms
Sodium:		1 mg
Exchanges:		1 fruit

Here's another topping recipe you can try. It can be used as a free food.

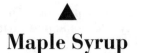

Maple Syrup

1¼ cups cold water
1 Tbsp. cornstarch
Artificial liquid sweetener—equal to 1 cup sugar
1 tsp. maple flavoring
⅛ tsp. salt

Combine ingredients in a saucepan. Bring to boil. Serve hot or cold over pancakes or waffles. Stir before using.

Yield:	1½ cups	Serving size: ¼ cup
Per serving:		
Calories:		8
Carbohydrate:		2 gms
Sodium:		0
Exchanges:		up to ½ cup free

The following recipe for another syrup was recommended by a teenager who has diabetes.

▲

Apple Juice Syrup

1 12 oz. can frozen apple juice concentrate
12 oz. water (equivalent amount of juice)
2–3 Tbsp. cornstarch
1 tsp. vanilla
1 tsp. cinnamon

Dissolve juice in water. Heat until almost boiling. To avoid lumping, dissolve cornstarch in small amount of liquid before adding to the remaining heated mixture. Heat until mixture is thickened to a syrup consistency. Add vanilla and cinnamon.

Yield:	3 cups	Serving size: ¼ cup
Per serving:		
Calories:		66
Carbohydrate:		16 gm
Sodium:		158 mg
Exchanges:		1 fruit

Here is a great way to bake potatoes. The potatoes have a crispy crust and don't need any additional margarine or sour cream, thus eliminating any added fat.

▲

Quick Baked Potato

1 large baking potato
Melted margarine, just enough to brush each potato half
Paprika
Parmesan cheese

Cut potato in half, brush cut half with melted margarine. Sprinkle potato with paprika and Parmesan cheese. Place cut half down on oiled cookie sheet. Bake at 350° for 25 to 30 minutes until potato is fork tender.

Yield:	2 servings	Serving size: ½ potato
Per serving:		
Calories:		84
Carbohydrate:		16 gms
Protein:		1 gm
Fat:		1 gm
Sodium:		38 mg
Exchanges:		1 starch/bread

This recipe can be used as a cream soup substitute that you can use in your favorite casserole recipe.

▲

Creamed Soup Mix

2 cups instant nonfat dry milk powder
¾ cup cornstarch
½ cup instant, low sodium chicken bouillon
2 Tbsp. dried onion flakes
1 tsp. dried, crushed basil
1 tsp. dried, crushed thyme
½ tsp. pepper

Combine all the ingredients. Mix and store in an airtight container. When you are ready to use, combine ⅓ cup of the mix with 1 ¼ cups water in a saucepan. Cook and stir until thickened. If you want to use the mix in place of cream of celery soup, add ¼ cup chopped celery; for mushroom soup, add ¼ cup chopped fresh mushrooms.

Yield:	3 cups mix (Equivalent to 9 10-oz. can soup)
Serving size:	⅓ cup
Calories:	96
Carbohydrate:	18 gm
Protein:	5 gm
Fat:	trace
Sodium:	310 mg
Exchanges:	1 starch/bread

▲

Syrup for Hot or Cold Chocolate Drink

½ cup unsweetened cocoa
Artificial sweetener equal to ½ cup plus 2½ Tbsp. sugar
½ cup hot water
2 tsp. vanilla

In saucepan, combine cocoa, artificial sweetener, sugar, and water. Mix well. Cook over medium heat stirring constantly until mixture comes to boiling point. Stir in vanilla. Store syrup in jar in refrigerator. Add 1 to 2 Tbsp., or less if desired, to skim milk allowance to make hot or cold chocolate. This cannot be used as a topping since it has a bitter taste before being mixed with milk.

Yield:	12 servings	Serving size: 2 Tbsp.
Per serving		
Calories:	17	
Carbohydrate:	2 gms	
Protein:	1 gm	
Fat:	trace	
Sodium:	262 mg	
Exchanges:	free	

Kool-Aid Mix

1 pkg. Kool-Aid (don't add sugar)
2¼-4 tsp. granulated artificial sweetener

Mix ingredients. Use ½ tsp. or more as desired of the mix per one cup of water. The mixture can be sealed in a plastic bag for travel or camping.

Yield:	8 cups	Serving size: 1 cup

Per serving:
Calories: 4
Carbohydrate: 1 gm
Sodium: 1 mg
Exchanges: free

▲

Low-Calorie Lemonade

Put ¼ tsp. non-caloric liquid sweetener in 2 Tbsp. lemon juice. Add to 1 cup water. Add ice as desired.

Yield:	1 cup	Serving size: 1 cup

Per serving:
Calories: 8
Carbohydrate: 2 gms
Sodium: trace
Exchanges: free

The following recipes are from Camp Needlepoint (American Diabetes Association of Minnesota's camp for children with diabetes).

▲

Homemade Granola

4 cups uncooked oatmeal (quick type)
1 cup chopped peanuts (no skins)
½ cup Grape Nuts
½ cup bran (unprocessed, uncooked)
Sugar substitute to equal ¼ cup sugar
⅓ cup vegetable oil
½ cup wheat germ
½ cup raisins

Spread the oatmeal on a cookie sheet and heat in a 350° oven for 10 minutes. Combine all but the last two ingredients. Bake on an ungreased cookie sheet or pan for 20 minutes, stirring once to brown evenly. Allow mixture to cook in the oven. Add wheat germ and raisins. Refrigerate in glass jars or plastic containers. (Granulated sugar substitute was more acceptable than liquid sugar substitute in this product.)

Yield: 6½ cups (26 servings)	Serving size: ¼ cup
Per serving:	
Calories:	140
Carbohydrate:	15 gms
Protein:	5 gms
Fat:	7 gms
Sodium:	57 mg
Exchanges:	1 starch/bread, 1 fat

Gorp

1 cup salted peanuts
1 cup raisins
1 cup sunflower seeds
1 cup each cereal: bran, wheat, corn chex

Mix all the ingredients together for a tasty snack. Store in an airtight container.

Yield:　6⅔ cups (20 servings)　　Serving size: ⅓ cup

Per serving:
Calories:　　　　　　　116
Carbohydrate:　　　　　12 gms
Protein:　　　　　　　　4 gms
Fat:　　　　　　　　　　6 gms
Sodium:　　　　　　　　110 mg
Exchanges:　　　　　　　1 starch/bread, 1 fat

▲

Cocoa Mix

⅓ cup nonfat dry milk
2½ tsp. powdered unsweetened cocoa
⅔ tsp. granulated artificial sweetener

Mix ingredients thoroughly. For camping, seal in a plastic bag. Add ¾ cup hot or cold water to dry mix (approximately 6 Tbsp.)

Yield:　　　1 serving　　　Serving size: 1 cup

Per serving:
Calories:　　　　　　　93
Carbohydrate:　　　　　14 gms
Protein:　　　　　　　　9 gms
Fat:　　　　　　　　　　trace
Sodium:　　　　　　　　124 mg
Exchanges:　　　　　　　1 low-fat milk

The smunchie recipes are from the Mason Clinic, Seattle, Washington, and are also served at Camp Needlepoint.

▲

Banana Smunchies

2 cups peanut butter
2 cups ripe bananas, mashed
52 graham cracker squares

Mash very ripe bananas into a smooth paste. Mix in peanut butter. Chill well. Drop 2 Tbsp. onto one square graham cracker, cover with second graham cracker square. Freeze until ready to use.

Yield:	26 servings	Serving size: 1 smunchie

Per serving:
Calories:	188
Carbohydrate:	20 gms
Protein:	7 gms
Fat:	11 gms
Sodium:	118 mg
Exchanges:	1 starch/bread
	1 med. fat meat, 1 fat

▲

Chocolate Smunchies

1 pkg. sugar-free chocolate pudding mix
2 cups nonfat milk
3 cups peanut butter
70 graham cracker squares

Mix chocolate pudding according to directions on package using nonfat milk. Cool thoroughly. Mix peanut butter with pudding. Drop 1 Tbsp. onto 1 square graham cracker. Place low-calorie whipped topping on top of the pudding/peanut butter mixture, cover with second graham cracker square. Freeze until ready to use.

Yield: 35 servings	Serving size: 1 smunchie

Per serving:
Calories:	200
Carbohydrate:	17 gms
Protein:	8 gms
Fat:	12 gms
Sodium:	142 mg
Exchanges:	1 starch/bread
	1 med. fat meat, 1 fat

These recipes are for the holiday foods included in the menus in Chapter 37.

▲

Spicy Tomato Cocktail

3 cups tomato juice
2 Tbsp. lemon juice
½ tsp sugar
¼ tsp. celery salt
½ tsp. Worcestershire sauce
6 lemon slices (optional)

Combine juice and seasonings. Chill. Garnish with lemon slice.

Yield:	6 servings	Serving Size: ½ cup
Calories:		28
Carbohydrate:		6 gm
Protein:		1 gm
Fat:		0
Sodium:		292 mg
Exchanges:		1 vegetable

▲

Cauliflower Supreme

1 large head cauliflower
1-1½ cups boiling water
2 cups seeded or seedless grapes
¼ cup slivered toasted almonds
1 tsp. salt

Break off each floret of the cauliflower, then slice lengthwise into slices ¼" thick. Simmer in boiling water in a covered skillet for 5 minutes or until tender. Drain. Fold in green grapes and almonds. Serve immediately.

Yield:	6 servings	Serving size: 1 cup

Per serving:
Calories:	83
Carbohydrate:	12 gms
Protein:	2 gms
Fat:	4 gms
Sodium:	390 mg
Exchanges:	½ fruit, 1 vegetable, 1 fat

▲

Cranberry-Celery Salad

1 envelope sugar-free gelatin (strawberry or cherry)
1 cup boiling water
1 Tbsp. lemon juice
1 cup coarsely ground cranberries
1 cup chopped celery
½ cup cold water

Add boiling water to gelatin. Stir until dissolved. Add cold water. Chill until partly set. Add lemon juice, chopped cranberries, and celery. Pour into decorative mold. Chill until set. Serve on lettuce.

Yield:	6 servings	Serving size: ⅙ of the mold

Per serving:
Calories:	20
Carbohydrate:	5 gms
Protein:	trace
Fat:	trace
Sodium:	22 mg
Exchanges:	1 serving = free
	3 servings = 1 fruit

▲

Low-Cal Pumpkin Pie

1 16 oz. can solid pumpkin
1 13 oz. can evaporated skim milk
1 egg OR
¼ cup Eggbeaters
½ cup Bisquick
1 Tbsp. sugar
8 pkg. artificial sweetener OR
1 Tbsp. liquid artificial sweetener
2 tsp. pumpkin pie spice
2 tsp. vanilla

Heat oven to 350°. Spray liquid spray shortening (e.g., Pam) in 9" pie plate. Blend all ingredients 1–2 minutes. Pour mixture into pie pan and bake 50 minutes.

Yield:	8 servings	Serving size: ⅛ of 9" pie
Per serving:		
Calories:		112
Carbohydrate:		18 gm
Protein:		6 gm
Fat:		2 gm
Sodium:		168 mg
Exchanges:		1 starch/bread, ½ fat

▲

Baked Pumpkin Pie

1 9" pie shell, unbaked
¼ cup sugar
½ tsp. cinnamon
½ tsp. ginger
½ tsp. nutmeg
pinch of cloves
1 cup canned pumpkin
1 tsp. vanilla

1 cup evaporated skim milk
½ tsp. orange rind
2 egg whites, slightly beaten
2½ Tbsp. brandy

Preheat oven to 450°. Combine all ingredients in large bowl and mix thoroughly. Pour into baked pie shell. Bake at 450° for 10 minutes, and then bake at 325° for 45 minutes or until knife inserted in filling comes out clean.

Yield:	8 servings	Serving size: ⅛ of 9" pie
Calories:		199
Carbohydrate:		22 gm
Protein:		5 gm
Fat:		8 gm
Sodium:		192 mg
Exchanges:		1½ starch/bread, 1½ fat

▲

Sparkling Sugar-Free Punch

½ cup granulated artificial sweetener
1½ cups water
2 cups low-calorie cranberry juice
2 cups pineapple juice
1 cup orange juice
1 28 oz. bottle sugar free ginger ale

Combine artificial sweetener and water in saucepan. Bring to a boil; cool. Pour chilled juices into large punch bowl and add cooled sweetener mixture. Add ginger ale just before serving.

Yield:	20 servings	Serving size: ½ cup
Calories:		24
Carbohydrate:		8 gm
Sodium:		2 mg
Exchanges:		1 serving = free
		2 servings = 1 fruit

▲

Green Beans Oregano

1 9 oz. pkg. frozen Italian green beans
1 cup diced tomato (about 1 medium tomato)
½ cup diced celery
¼ cup diced green pepper
2 Tbsp. chopped onion
¼ tsp. dried oregano leaves
⅓ cup water
4 lemon wedges

Combine all ingredients in a saucepan and bring to a boil. Separate beans with a fork. Reduce heat, cover and simmer 6 to 8 minutes, or until beans are tender-crisp. Serve with lemon wedges.

Yield:	4 servings	Serving size: ½ cup
Calories:		24
Carbohydrate:		5 gm
Protein:		2 gm
Sodium:		11 mg
Exchanges:		1 vegetable

Flaming Cherries Jubilee

1 can (16 oz.) water-packed or juice-packed dark cherries
2 tsp. cornstarch
1 tsp. sugar
½ tsp. artificial liquid sweetener
¼ cup cherry brandy
red food coloring
¼ cup Cherry Kirsch (to flame)

Drain cherries. Add water to cherry liquid to make ¾ cup. In saucepan, combine cornstarch and sugar; blend in cherry liquid. Cook and stir until thickened. Add cherries, liquid sweetener, cherry brandy, and a few drops food coloring. Serve hot.

To Flame: Slowly heat Cherry Kirsch in a small saucepan for a few minutes. DO NOT BOIL. Light with match and pour over cherries. (Be sure cherry mixture is hot.)

Yield: 4 servings	Serving size: ¾ cup
Per serving:	
Calories:	61
Carbohydrate:	14 gms
Protein:	trace
Sodium:	2 mg
Exchanges:	1 fruit

The cherry sauce also may be used to garnish other desserts. Spoon sauce over ½ cup vanilla ice cream (1 starch/bread and 2 fat exchanges) or over 1½" cube sponge cake (1 starch/bread exchange.)

▲

Wiggley Easter Shapes

1 envelope sugar-free gelatin

Prepare gelatin using fruit juice in place of half of the water called for. Do not add any water. Pour into a small rectangular pan and refrigerate until set. Use Easter cookie cutters and cut into Easter shapes.

Yield:	4 servings	Serving size: ½ cup
Per serving:		
Calories:		56
Carbohydrate:		14 gms
Sodium:		9 mg
Exchanges:		1 fruit

▲

Bunny Salad

Place crisp lettuce leaf on a plate. Place two chilled, unsweetened pear halves upside down on top of lettuce. Make 2 bunnies, using narrow end for the face.

Eyes: 4 cloves
Nose: 2 pimiento
Ears: 4 blanched whole almonds
Tail: Cottage cheese formed into 2 balls

Yield: 2 bunnies   Serving size: 2 bunnies

Per serving:
Calories: 56
Carbohydrate: 14 gms
Sodium: 1 mg
Exchanges: 1 fruit

▲

Potato Soufflé

1½ pounds potatoes, peeled and cubed
1 Tbsp. margarine
1 onion, chopped
1 cup fresh mushrooms, chopped
¼ cup grated Parmesan
Dash of pepper
3 egg yolks
6 egg whites

Preheat oven to 325°. Grease a 2-quart souffle dish or casserole. Sprinkle 1 Tbsp. Parmesan on bottom and sides; set aside. Cook potatoes in water about 10 minutes until soft. Drain and mash with ½ Tbsp. margarine. Saute onions in ½ Tbsp. margarine for 2 minutes. Add mushrooms and saute. Combine potatoes and vegetables. Beat egg yolks one at a time into mixture. Beat egg whites until stiff but not dry. Fold egg whites into potato mixture. Transfer to prepared dish. Bake 45–50 minutes. Serve immediately.

Yield: 8 servings   Serving size: 1 cup

Calories: 155
Carbohydrate: 19 gm
Protein: 6 gm
Fat: 5 gm
Sodium: 140 mg
Exchanges: 1 starch/bread, 1 fat

▲

Carrot Orange Toss

2 oranges, diced
2 cups grated carrots
2 Tbsp. honey
1 tsp. lemon juice
½ cup raisins

Combine all ingredients. Chill. Serve on lettuce cups.

Yield:	8 servings	Serving size: ½ cup
Per serving:		
Calories:		88
Carbohydrate:		21 gms
Protein:		1 gm
Sodium:		31 mg
Exchanges:		1 fruit, 1 vegetable

▲

Strawberry Trifle

½ large or 1 small angel food cake
3 oz. box sugar-free strawberry gelatin
10 oz. Lite frozen strawberries, thawed
2 bananas, large
2 9-oz. boxes instant sugar-free vanilla pudding
9 oz. Lite Cool Whip

Tear cake into bite-size pieces and place in bottom of ungreased 9"x13" pan. Dissolve gelatin in 1 cup boiling water—no cold water. Add strawberries and their juice to gelatin. Spoon evenly over cake pieces. Slice bananas on top and refrigerate while you prepare the pudding, which should be made with skim milk. Pour pudding over the bananas and top with Lite Cool Whip. Refrigerate 1 to 2 hours. Cut into squares to serve. (A pancake turner works great to serve.) Garnish with a slice of fresh strawberry, if available.

Yield:	15 servings	Serving size: 3" x 2-½"
Calories:		124
Carbohydrate:		23 gm
Protein:		3 gm
Fat:		3 gm
Sodium:		314 mg
Exchanges:		1 starch/bread
		½ fruit, ½ fat

Easter Sparkle Dessert

1 envelope lemon flavored sugar-free gelatin
1 envelope lime flavored sugar-free gelatin

Prepare the gelatin using the directions on the envelope of each package. Pour each flavor separately into a pie pan and place in the refrigerator to gel. As soon as the gelatin is set, take a sharp knife and cut into ½" cubes. Pile the cubes into a sherbet glass, alternating the lemon and lime. This dessert really sparkles!

Yield:	two 9" pie pans	Serving size: ½ cup
Per serving:		
Calories:		8
Carbohydrate:		2 gms
Sodium:		8 mg
Exchanges:		up to 1 cup, free

▲

Marshmallow Crispies

1 Tbsp. vegetable oil
40 large (or 4 cups miniature) marshmallows
4 cups crisp rice cereal

Grease large saucepan with cooking oil. Add marshmallows and melt over low heat; watch carefully. Quickly stir in cereal; mix well. With buttered spoon, press into greased 8 x 8 x 2-inch pan. Cut into 25 squares.

Yield:	25 squares	Serving size: 1 square

Per serving:
Calories: 60
Carbohydrate: 15 gms
Protein: trace
Fat: trace
Sodium: 39 mg
Exchanges: 1 fruit

▲

Angel Macaroons

16 oz. one-step angel food cake mix
½ cup sugar-free strawberry flavored carbonated beverage
2 tsp. vanilla or almond extract
2 cups unsweetened shredded coconut
½ cup chopped walnuts

Cover baking sheet with aluminum foil. In large mixing bowl, beat the cake mix together with the carbonated beverage and vanilla on low speed for 30 seconds, then at medium speed for 1 minute, scraping sides of bowl. Fold in coconut and nuts. Drop by teaspoonfuls onto foil-lined baking sheet, 2 inches apart. Bake at 350° for 10 to 12 minutes. Slide foil onto cooling rack. Cool. Store in airtight containers.

Yield:	60	Serving size: 2 cookies

Per serving:
Calories: 98
Carbohydrate: 14 gm
Protein: 2 gm
Fat: 4 gm
Sodium: 112 mg
Exchanges: 1 starch/bread, 1 fat

▲ REFERENCES ▲

Section One:

Monk A. *Convenience Food Facts. Help for Planning Quick, Healthy, and Convenient Meals*. DCI/CHRONIMED Publishing, Minneapolis, MN, 1991.

Pennington JAT. *Bowes and Church's Food Values of Portions Commonly Used*. Fifteenth Edition. JB Lippincott, Philadelphia, 1989.

United States Department of Agriculture, Human Nutrition Information Service. Composition of Foods. Agriculture Handbook 8 Series: 8-1 to 8-22, 1976-1990.

Section Two:

The American Dietetic Association, American Diabetes Association. *Ethnic and Regional Food Practices*. A Series—*Hmong American* (1992), *Jewish* (1989), *Mexican American* (1989), *Navajo* (1991), *Chinese American* (1990). American Dietetic Association, Chicago.

Cooper, N. *The Joy of Snacks*. DCI/CHRONIMED Publishing, Minneapolis, MN, 1991.

Franz MJ. *Fast Food Facts. Nutritive and Exchange Values for Fast-Food Restaurants*. DCI/CHRONIMED Publishing, Minneapolis, MN, 1993.

Kahn AP. Keeping Kosher. *Diabetes Self-Management* 1989; March/April:33–41.

Kittler PG, Sucher P. *Food and Culture in America*. Van Nostrand Reinhold, New York, 1989.

Monk A. *Convenience Food Facts. Help for Planning Quick, Healthy, and Convenient Meals*. DCI/CHRONIMED Publishing, Minneapolis, MN, 1991.

United States Department of Agriculture, Human Nutrition Information Service. Composition of Foods. Agriculture Handbook Numbers 8-19, 8-21, 1976-1990.

Warshaw HS. *The Restaurant Companion. A Guide to Healthier Eating Out.* Surrey Books, Chicago, 1990.

Addresses for freeze-dried camp food:

Alpine Aire PO, Box 926, Nevada City, CA 95959.

Mountain House, Oregon Freeze Dry Inc., PO Box 1048, Albany, OR 97321.

Section Three:

American Dietetic Association Position Paper. Use of nutritive and non-nutritive sweeteners. *J Am Diet Assoc* (in press).

Franz MJ, Cooper N. Meal planning: adding flexibility. In: Franz MJ, Etzwiler DD, Joynes JO, Hollander PA, eds. *Learning to Live Well with Diabetes.* DCI/CHRONIMED Publishing, Minneapolis, MN, 1991, pp. 305–320.

Franz MJ. Nutrition: the cornerstone. In: Franz MJ, Etzwiler DD, Joynes JO, Hollander PA, eds. *Learning to Live Well with Diabetes.* DCI/CHRONIMED Publishing, Minneapolis, MN, 1991, pp. 21–48.

Franz MJ, Hedding BK, Leitch G. *Opening the Door to Good Nutrition.* DCI/CHRONIMED Publishing, Minneapolis, MN, 1985.

MacRae NM. *Canning and Preserving Without Sugar.* Pacific Search Press, Seattle, WA, 1982.

Reader D, Franz MJ. *Pass the Pepper!* DCI/CHRONIMED Publishing, Minneapolis, MN, 1988.

Section Four:

A la Grecque, A la King, A la What? A Guide to Restaurant Terms. American Institute for Cancer Research Newsletter, Winter 1992.

Cooper NA. *The Joy of Snacks.* DCI/CHRONIMED Publishing, Minneapolis, MN, 1991.

Franz MJ. Alcohol and diabetes: part I. *Diabetes Spectrum* 1990; 3:136–144.

Franz MJ. Alcohol and diabetes: part II. *Diabetes Spectrum* 1990; 3:210–215.

Franz MJ. Fuel for exercise. *Diabetes Forecast* 1992; 46(10): 30–33.

Franz MJ, Cooper N. Meal planning: adding flexibility. In: Franz et al. *Learning to Live Well with Diabetes*. DCI/CHRONIMED Publishing, Minneapolis, MN, 1991, pp.305–320.

Franz MJ, Norstrom J. Exercise: the advantage is yours; clues for safe participation; the answer to improved blood glucose control. In: Franz et al. *Learning to Live Well with Diabetes*. DCI/CHRON-IMED Publishing, Minneapolis, MN, 1991, pp. 49–64.

Horton ES. Exercise and decreased risk of NIDDM. *N En J Med* 1991; 325:196–198.

Pearson J. Planes, trains, and automobiles: plan your way to a fun-filled vacation. *Living Well with Diabetes* 1991; Summer:15–16.

Roth H. *Guide to Low-Cholesterol Dining Out*. Penguin Books, New York, 1990.

Sane T, Koivisto VA, Nikkanen P, Pelkonen R. Adjusting of insulin doses of diabetic patients during long distance flights. *Br Med J* 1990; 301:421–422.

United States Department of Agriculture. Meal Pattern Requirements and Offer Versus Serve Manual. USDA/Food and Nutrition Service FNS-265, 1990.

Warshaw HS. *The Restaurant Companion. A Guide to Healthier Eating Out*. Surrey Books, Chicago, 1990.

▲ INDEX ▲